PENGUIN BOOKS

7 DAYS TO STRIP FAT FOREVER

Shane Bilsborough is a co-director of the lifestyle management consulting company, B Personal, where he works as a nutritionist, personal trainer and research scientist. Shane has a Master's degree in Human Nutrition from Deakin University in Melbourne, Australia, and has written many articles on health, diet and the impact of physical fitness on weight, in particular fat weight. Following the success of his first book, *The Fat-Stripping Diet*, Shane is a regular public speaker and also works as a weight-loss consultant online. He lives in Melbourne with his wife Fiona.

Shane can be contacted at www.bpersonal.com.au.

D0470096

SHANE BILSBOROUGH

7days to
strip fat
forever

PENGUIN BOOKS

The fat grams shown in the tables on pages 161–170 were sourced from Nutrition for Life *by Catherine Saxelby, Hardie Grant Books, Melbourne, 1996.*

Penguin Books

Published by the Penguin Group
Penguin Books Australia Ltd
250 Camberwell Road, Camberwell, Victoria 3124, Australia
Penguin Books Ltd
80 Strand, London WC2R 0RL, England
Penguin Putnam Inc.
375 Hudson Street, New York, New York 10014, USA
Penguin Books Canada Limited
10 Alcorn Avenue, Toronto, Ontario, Canada M4V 3B2
Penguin Books (NZ) Ltd
Cnr Rosedale and Airborne Roads, Albany, Auckland, New Zealand
Penguin Books (South Africa) (Pty) Ltd
24 Sturdee Avenue, Rosebank, Johannesburg 2196, South Africa
Penguin Books India (P) Ltd
11, Community Centre, Panchsheel Park, New Delhi 110 017, India

First published by Penguin Books Australia Ltd 2002

5 7 9 10 8 6

Cover design by David Altheim, Penguin Design Studio
Text design by Susannah Low, Penguin Design Studio
Cover photograph by Tim de Neefe
Typeset in 11/16 pt Minion by Post Pre-Press Group, Brisbane, Queensland
Printed and bound in Australia by McPherson's Printing Group, Maryborough, Victoria

National Library of Australia
Cataloguing-in-Publication data:

Bilsborough, Shane.
7 days to strip fat forever.

Includes index.
ISBN 0 14 300022 5.

1. Reducing diets. 2. Low-fat diet. 3. Low-calorie diet.
I. Title.

613.25

www.penguin.com.au

CONTENTS

INTRODUCTION

When you understand how your body works you are empowered to take control of your life and work with the body's processes, rather than fighting them. This leads to the desired results of weight loss and self-confidence, and you become inspirational to others. In this book you will learn how to keep fat off your body permanently and how to combine this with achieving optimum health and energy levels.

The enormous response to my first book, *The Fat-Stripping Diet*, saw it become a number one bestseller. It made me realise that people were at last ready to hear the truth about fat loss. I realised that people wanted to know not just what to eat but how to eat to lose weight.

The new fat-loss plan

We are all overeating, but we really don't need to. With a few simple tricks, you can eat very well and still lose weight. The new 7×7 Fat-Reducing Plan is successful, safe and extremely easy to follow. The diet works on the principles followed by many Asian cultures, and cultures that are lean and disease-free. It also recognises recent breakthroughs made by scientific studies on reducing the 'energy density' of our food. By following the new 7×7 Fat-Reducing Plan you will not overeat, allowing your body easier access to your fat stores. But you will not go hungry either.

The Plan extends and further implements the revolutionary principles brought about by the Fat-Stripping Diet – it keeps your fat intake to a level where you can use body fat for energy, and reduces the energy density of your meals. It works on the consumption of seven meals a day, seven days a week. This is a lot of eating! But in seven days you can trigger the avalanche of fat loss. Taking progressive small steps – day by day and week by week – and understanding what these small steps are doing to your body helps you to achieve your desired results in both the short term and the long term.

The results from following this plan have been awesome. One man, Chris, who had tried almost every weight-loss method and failed, plummeted from 119 kilograms to 98 kilograms in just fifteen weeks. Chris lost the majority of his weight from fat, not muscle and water, and has been able to keep this weight off for well over six months. Chris is just one of many success stories. Some of our other clients have wanted to lose 4 or 5 kilograms, and they too have achieved this with relative ease. Remember that this is fat loss, not muscle loss.

Healthy bodies – inside and out

Hundreds of people have asked me to write a diet for them that would not only reduce their weight, but would help them with heart disease. As time went on, more and more people approached me about this important issue, especially busy corporate people. Here I have written a separate diet and lifestyle program for anyone suffering from risk factors such as high cholesterol, blood pressure or stress, or who is very overweight. The 7×6 Heart Plan is very simple to follow, easy to understand, and works hand in hand with the 7×7 Fat-Reducing Plan. It allows people to lose weight while also improving their health. Once you have reduced your risk factors by following the 7×6 Heart Plan, you can follow the 7×7 Fat-Reducing Plan. For the many people who have requested these diets, here they are! For those who don't have any of the symptoms of heart disease, don't neglect this chapter. The scary thing is that most of us already have the earliest signs of heart disease and have probably had them for a while – yet don't even know it. These early signs have been found in the blood vessels of children as young as five years old.

The realities of fat loss

In *7 Days to Strip Fat Forever* I have refined one of most empowering tools that have been used by many people to show how bad too much fat is: the Bilsborough Fat Cost Chart. This chart finally allows you to see the cost of fat. Fat takes a lot of time to walk off and with this chart you can see exactly how long and how far it will take you. Imagine knowing that the average American or Australian man or woman needs to walk for 100 minutes and 130 minutes respectively just to use up the fat they eat every day! In coming to terms with this you are coming to terms with why fat gain is so easy; and why fat loss is so hard if you don't understand how it works.

High protein vs low carbohydrate

In many hundreds of emails people requested information about the high-protein/low-carbohydrate diets. Many people tell me how they are trying to balance their insulin in order to lose weight. Please folks, you are trying to be too scientific. You are focusing on the wrong aspect of your health! Losing fat is all about reducing fat and increasing fibre in your diet. Nothing more, nothing less. The same people who tell you to balance insulin have probably told you to cut out carbohydrates. They have also probably forgotten to mention some side effects. Well, try this. It is well established that high-protein/low-carbohydrate diets are linked to osteoporosis, heart disease, muscle wasting, dehydration, decreases in the contraction rate of the heart, heart arrhythmias and sudden death. Sounds shocking? It is, and I wonder how many people are at risk and don't know it.

Long-term success

The results that people achieved on the Fat-Stripping Diet were absolutely outstanding, especially in the long-term. I knew they would be. We have recorded well over three thousand cases of people who have lost more than 8 kilograms and kept it off. Well done, and I'm sure there are many more. Thank you for all the emails. Here is just one letter I would like to share with you:

Dear Shane,

I have tried many diets and read many books on how to lose weight. Until I read The Fat-Stripping Diet *I was never able to keep weight off. When I found out how much time it took to work off fat I nearly fell off my chair. Bingo! Exactly what I needed to know. All the garbage I read about balancing my insulin with protein and cutting out carbohydrates was just ridiculous. I'm a mother of three and there needs to be pasta and rice on the table. As I've learnt, the secret is keeping the fat such as the olive oil and cheese very low! In eight months since I read your book, I am no longer on a diet, but a new lifestyle. I have lost nearly 15 kilograms and it has stayed off. The impact that the book has had on my family has been wonderful too. My husband and my children are still following your eating plan and they all look and feel so much better.*

Thanking you kindly
Mrs P Richards

Accessible fat loss

Obviously, much of the research behind this book is quite technical, so when faced with how best to advise readers, I have opted for the most practical advice for the average person. This is especially the case with the information on exercise, which was compiled with the help of many fitness professionals and exercise physiologists. Exercise is an integral part of good health and increasing your fat loss, if done correctly. Finding the time to exercise is your challenge; awesome health and fat loss are your rewards. Once again the focus is on a period of seven days of being active.

7 Days to Strip Fat Forever will provide you with more tools to lose fat for good as well as keeping you in good health. There are many thousands of people who are keeping weight off. They are keeping it off in the long term and living fulfilling, changed, healthy lives. Put your mind to it and I know you too will achieve your weight-loss goals. Whether it is 4 kilograms or 15 kilograms, be patient! It may take you a little longer to lose weight than someone else. Aim for the short term and look long-term. When following *7 Days to Strip Fat Forever* surround yourself with positive people and be positive yourself. I am a strong believer that we can achieve anything if we truly believe we can. This is certainly true with fat loss.

Eat well, live well – and good luck.

CHAPTER 1

HOW CAN I STRIP FAT?

Key messages for this chapter

YOU WILL DISCOVER:

- why the human population is becoming more obese
- how easy it is to store fat
- why you feel that you put on weight all of a sudden
- that to lose weight you have to reduce your fat intake

Just tell me how to lose weight!

I am sure that by now most of you reading this book have heard it all. There is so much rubbish written about how to lose weight that most people either are incredibly confused or have just given up in frustration. As a qualified sports nutritionist, personal trainer and public speaker on weight loss, the most common plea I hear is, 'Just tell me how to lose weight!'

I know that when people say this they want to know not only how to lose weight but also how to keep it off. So we're actually talking about fat, not just weight. People want to keep fat off in the long term, not just look good for a short period of time. Most people think that they can lose weight by not eating, or by severe food restriction, but as soon as they start to eat normally again they just pile this weight back on. People are sick of regaining weight and yo-yoing. Hence the plea changes to: 'Just tell me how to lose *fat* and keep it off for good!'

Boom time

The 1980s was a time when humans generally grew larger and stored more fat than they had previously. The predictions for the nineties and the twenty-first century showed that we were heading for chronic proportions of overweight and obese populations. Even once thin races of people started to become overweight and large races were getting larger. My own father, who once lived on the island of Sri Lanka, registered barely

49 kilograms on the scales while living in his island hometown. In the years after his migration to Australia he tipped the scales at a whopping 100 kilograms, as a result of embracing the lifestyle of Western society.

Weight-loss industries

Recent decades have seen the billion-dollar weight-loss industry move into full swing with many new and ingenious weight-loss options. There have been low-fat foods, low-fat milk, diet drinks and artificial sweeteners. People believed that they could eat as much low-fat food as they wanted, but they ended up consuming even more fat than they otherwise would have. Then there's been the boom of weight-loss products that falsely promises cures for cellulite and fat. These products promise spot reduction and amazing fat-burning results, made with secret recipes from Amazon tribes, or rare herbs found only in the jungles of Africa. I have witnessed a salesman tell my friend that by rubbing a particular hot weight-loss herb on her skin, her fat would ooze from inside her to the skin where she could scoop it up and get rid of it. Needless to say I was absolutely stunned, but more so by how willing my friend was to purchase the product.

Many misconceptions about weight loss have been promoted. And no effort is considered too great in the quest to lose fat. People have run around the streets or power-walked with garbage bags under their clothing. Some even thought that by running while wearing layered, thick woollen clothing during 40-degree heat, fat would ooze out of their bodies. There were others who simply thought that not eating was the safest and most effective ploy for weight loss.

The origins of body fat

During hunter–gatherer times, when food was in a short supply people survived because they had the ability to store energy for 'lean times'. Of course, thousands of years ago this was a key element needed in order to survive. If you didn't have the genes that allowed your body to store fat, then your family tree would have stopped many years ago. Some people argue that we should eat the way our hunter–gatherer ancestors did, which means plenty of meat, leaves, seeds, fruits and vegetables. The problem here is that meat caught in prehistoric times would have been much leaner than today, and contained less bad fat and more good fats (see pages 23–25). Animals wouldn't have been pumped full of growth accelerators and antibiotics, as they are now.

What people forget is that these ancestors had no ready supply of food, no twenty-four-hour supermarket next door. They had to expend the energy equivalent of a half-marathon just to catch their food, and when food wasn't abundant they went for days living off their fat stores.

As time progresses, the human population becomes larger and larger, particularly in opulent Western societies, such as Australia, the United Kingdom and the United States. Now we live in a time that scientists refer to as obesogenic or obese-forming. We are putting on weight because, among other things, we eat too much fat. High-fat and low-fibre diets are a common factor in weight and fat gain, and also in nearly all disease. We are eating far too much fat (from far too much food) for our bodies to burn up. This results in higher rates of heart disease and early deaths that many health professionals say could be avoided. Our children are also getting fatter and fatter, and obesity in children under ten is increasingly common.

So why are we getting fatter?

Reports from around the world have shown that we are eating about 2–3 per cent less fat than we were five years ago. Statistics show that in the USA, UK and Australia, the average man eats about 100 grams of fat each day and an average woman eats 70 grams of fat. However, while people claim to be eating less fat, scientific studies show that many people under-report their fat intake by 30–70 per cent when they fill out nutrition surveys. This means actual fat intake could be 123–180 grams for men per day and 83–100 grams for women. This is a huge amount of fat and too much for our bodies to burn up.

The body will use a minimum of fat each day to provide energy for its metabolism. For women, this means the body will burn up to 41 grams of fat per day and for men, 60 grams per day. Your metabolic rate is responsible for:

- keeping your heart beating and pumping blood around the body

- your breathing
- breaking down food, transporting and storing it
- making new cells and removing old ones
- filtering blood through your kidneys.

Any fat you eat over this 41 or 60 grams will be stored around the body as excess fat. This means that we are still eating much more fat than we need. A daily excess of 25 grams for women and 40 grams for men results in a yearly fat gain of nearly 9 kilograms and 14 kilograms respectively.

BUILD-UP OF FAT STORAGE

TIME	MEN	WOMEN
1 week	280 g	175 g
1 month	1.12 kg	700 g
1 year	13.4 kg	8.4 kg

In the Western world today we rarely suffer from hunger or famines. What is the point in having a genetic system that easily stores fat when you live less than a block away from a fish and chip shop or an 'all you can eat' restaurant? Recently statistics have tried to solve the paradox of overnutrition. Is the fact that we have such easy access to food working against us? The fact that we can eat as much food as we want may lead to an earlier death. Obesity and high-fat, low-fibre diets are an enormous problem for the Western world.

The more fat we eat, the more fat we store

There is no limit to fat storage. Our fat cells just keep on getting larger and can enlarge twenty times in diameter and two to three thousand times their volume to store fat. They can even increase in number. We have the ability to make fat cells until the day we die. This is because when we fill up our fat cells, the body can make new ones. This is basic fat physiology.

Scientists used to think there were specific times when fat cell numbers increased: during rapid growth spurts, in early infancy from one to two years, during early adolescence from twelve to fourteen years, and during pregnancy. (This is called lipogenesis.) But scientific evidence now shows that fat cell numbers can increase at any time, once existing fat cells are full.

It's not all bad news, however. Fat cells can also be starved of fat and hence made to shrivel up and die. By lowering the amount of fat that you eat, fat storage is decreased. The human body doesn't like to have cells hanging around doing nothing, so with time these cells get smaller and smaller. In fact when you lose fat, most of your fat cells shrink and eventually die. This process is called apoptosis. Following the eating plan in this book (see Chapter 3) will help you lose fat and fat cells.

Energy density

'Energy density' is the new buzzword in fat loss. In the Western world there are three main problems that result in weight gain. We eat too much fat, we eat too much food and we eat very little fibre. The more fat we eat, the less fibre we are likely to eat, and hence the larger the 'energy density' of a meal. The message from health professionals is to decrease the amount of fat we eat, and increase the amount of fibrous foods, found especially in fruit and vegetables. In 2002 people eat about 10 per cent more food than they did ten years ago. This means we are still eating too much fat and too much food. The energy density of our food is very high.

Dr David Cameron-Smith, senior lecturer at Deakin University and an expert on nutrition, genetics and obesity prevention, says, 'The message is to reduce the amount of fat we eat, reduce the amount of food we eat, and this in turn reduces the energy density of our meals.'

Cutting down the amount of fat we eat each day is the first and most vital step in weight and fat loss. In simple terms, if the average man cut his fat intake from 100 grams per day to 50 grams, he would save 1890 kJ of energy each day. This cuts down the amount of energy he eats each day from 11 000 kJ to 9110 kJ. If the average woman cut her fat intake down from 70 grams to 35 grams per day she would save 1323 kJ each day and reduce her energy eaten from 7500 kJ to 6177 kJ. The weight loss in a year would be over 12–15 kilograms, due to a reduction in the energy density of the daily meals. Reducing the amount of fat you eat reduces the energy density of your meals.

Making better low-fat choices
Many lower-fat products have higher amounts of protein and sugar than their full-fat versions. People need to make better

low-fat choices, by reading the labels on the packaging carefully. It makes little sense cutting down fat and then increasing sugar. A little sugar in your diet does no harm, but the more sugar you eat the less fibre you will eat. All this does is increase the energy density of the meal. This is especially true for low-fat products that are sweet. Most of us make an effort to buy low-fat alternatives, but research indicates that many people replace high-fat products with the wrong low-fat ones. 'Lite' or 'reduced-fat' labelling doesn't necessarily mean it's low in fat or you can eat twice as much. In examining some popular yoghurt products on the market, I came across a good example of the topic of energy density.

READING THE LABELS

ALL 200-GRAM SERVES	ENERGY DENSITY (kJ)	PROTEIN (g)	FAT (g)	CARBO-HYDRATES (sugar) (g)
Natural, unsweetened yoghurt, full-fat	720	9	9.6	12.2
Reduced-fat yoghurt 1 (bad choice)	827	9.8	5.9	26.2
Reduced-fat yoghurt 2 (good choice)	315	8.6	0.2	9.7

The three yoghurts I chose were a regular-fat variety and two reduced-fat varieties. As you can see, the second low-fat yoghurt had low amounts of sugar and fat, and hence low energy, or energy density (315 kJ). Choosing this yoghurt is a good low-fat choice. The first reduced-fat yoghurt had a little less fat than the full-fat variety but over double the amount of sugar. The energy density of this yoghurt is higher than the full-fat variety (827 kJ compared to 720 kJ). This is a clear example of making a bad choice with low-fat foods.

The problem is when people eat three to four of these low-fat yoghurts in a day. Yes, they are very low in fat, but the ideal choice is to substitute low fat for a piece of fibre-containing fruit. Another classic example of a high-energy-density meal is the traditional steak and vegetable meal. Most people have their plate covered by a large piece of meat and a small amount of vegetables, followed by a dessert. We need to understand that we are overeating protein such as red meat and this too can lead to weight gain. To change this into a low-energy-density meal, fill the plate with vegetables, cut down the size of the meat, and eat fruit salad for dessert. To further cut down the energy density, reduce the amount you eat. By following this simple, unconventional procedure, you can reduce the energy density of the meal by nearly 50–60 per cent and help reduce weight gain.

What is fat?

We know that fat surrounds living tissue such as muscles and organs to provide cushioning and padding to areas such as your eye sockets, fingers and toes, heels of your feet, joints and specific areas such as your back. Fat is known in scientific circles as adipose tissue. This adipose tissue is the storage site for fat that we eat. It has a honeycomb structure of large spherically shaped cells, like balloons, that has been described by some scientists as 'the ultimate in biological bubble wrap'.

Although the storage of excess fat in adipose tissue means that many people are overweight, some fat is essential for the human body. Essential fatty acids are found in olive oil and sunflower oil, among other products, and we need these fats for energy for our bodies to function properly (see pages 23–25). These fats are not included in our daily fat balance of 41 grams for women and 60 grams for men, because when eaten in small amounts they don't get converted to body fat.

NO BODY FAT

Congenital generalised lipodystrophy is a rare recessive genetic condition. People with this syndrome have literally no adipose tissue, so fat has no place to be stored in the body. In other words they are born without body fat. These people also have very limited muscle on their body. They never reach sexual maturity and, in the case of women, they remain infertile. Their body fat levels are too low for them to reproduce.

It is so easy to store fat. It costs the body only 3 per cent of the incoming energy to undertake this process. For example, if you ate a 150 gram block of cheese (50 grams of fat), 48.5 grams would be stored as fat. It is very easy to store fat but much harder to work it off.

Staying trim

No-one is exempt from storing fat. If you are thin now, don't take it for granted that you will stay like that forever. Fat can be stored almost imperceptibly and then often it seems that you've put on weight all of a sudden. Younger people or sportspeople who don't have a weight problem now may have one later on. If you are fortunate enough not to be overweight, then I suggest that you start looking at putting some good eating and/or exercising plans into action immediately.

People often tell me that they gained weight all of a sudden, without warning. The weight gain always seems to 'sneak up', but fat accumulates ever so easily bit by bit over many years. You don't notice weight gain when it's slowing accumulating. Of course, during this time you feel that you can eat what you want. Putting on 30 grams here or storing 50 grams there would hardly be noticeable, but overeating during a week may result in 250 grams of fat being stored. Fat cells are found all over the body, so over a short period of time fat gain may not be noticed. Fat is not very heavy when compared to muscle so it may not even register on the scales.

Whether you want to lose 5 kilograms or 15 kilograms, the process of fat loss is the same. The point is never to take for granted that you can eat what you like without becoming overweight. Don't wait until you gain weight to do something about it. This is particularly important for younger people, who have the advantage of having a faster metabolism and still have time to develop good lifestyle habits.

Fat is a problem not just for the people carrying a little bit more weight than they need; it's also a problem for the thinner people who will gain weight in the future. You establish the patterns of your lifestyle now, so it's important to restrict the fat consumption in your diet. When this becomes second nature, most of the hard work has been done. The eating plan in this book is for everyone, for people who want to shed a few kilograms and for those who want to lose 10 or 20 kilograms.

Obesity

Peter, a former client of ours at B Personal, ate himself to obesity. His busy lifestyle and very long working hours meant that he always ate on the run, at restaurants and rarely at home. Most foods eaten out are fatty foods. He very rarely thought about healthy eating until one day his scale weight registered 117 kilograms. We calculated Peter's dietary energy intake and in particular his energy from fat. He ate a massive 256 grams of fat every day. This means he would store 196 grams of fat every day (256 – 60).

As the table on page 14 shows, this extremely high-fat intake can make a person of reasonable weight bulk up. Peter's high-fat intake means that his fat cells would have enlarged, and his body would have produced new cells to cope with this fat storage.

PETER'S FAT ACCUMULATION

WEEK	FAT STORED
1	1.3 kg
2	2.7 kg
3	4 kg
4	5.3 kg
8	6.6 kg
15	13 kg
52	26 kg

As a person moves from being overweight to being obese, the body develops many risk factors. These include hypertension, high cholesterol, heart failure and diabetes. Renal disease, gallstone disease, osteoarthritis, cancer and joint injuries are also very common. This litany of health problems is a very real threat to overweight and obese people.

There are many reasons why people put on weight and in particular fat weight. Some people blame themselves for their excess weight gain, but sometimes genetics plays a large role. Science is always striving to determine why people become overweight and how much of a part the genetic pattern of our parents and grandparents plays. It seems that our genes are partly responsible, but what we eat, how much we eat and how active we are play just as important a role. In a recent study, six infants of lean mothers and twelve of overweight mothers were studied to see how much energy they used. This study followed the weight gain of infants from nine days to one year.

Of infants born to overweight mothers, 50 per cent became overweight after one year. These same infants used 20.7 per cent less energy after three months than the infants of lean mothers. In a mass study of 673 twins, with pairs reared together and apart, it was concluded that environmental factors contributed to about 30 per cent of weight gain. We have seen overweight people whose parents and grandparents were overweight, or even obese, follow sensible lifestyle practices and remain lean. This shows that the vast majority of people can lose weight, and in particular fat weight, despite their genetics.

Regardless of the reasons for putting on weight, the consequences of weight gain can cut short a person's life, or at least make life very uncomfortable and difficult. The stresses on the joints, especially the back and knees, start to take a toll. The overweight person who tackles this issue head-on can reduce many risk factors and live a happier, longer life.

Real people losing real fat

The problem is that fat gets stored as fat, and the only way to reduce fat in the body is to reduce the actual consumption of fat in your diet and be more physically active. With the 7×7 Fat-Reducing Plan, I recommend that women consume less than 41 grams per day and men consume less that 60 grams for effective fat loss (see pages 5–6). This eating plan follows the same principles as the Fat-Stripping Diet, which were developed in my first book, but here they are taken to a new level.

In my dietary research, I base my eating plans for both men and women on the following daily intake. The 21 per cent fat comes only from plant oils, not animal fats. It's important to state here that the 7×7 Fat-Reducing Plan is not a high-carbohydrate diet; it simply has a higher percentage of plant-derived carbohydrates than proteins.

IDEAL DAILY INTAKE

Carbohydrates (plant food)	55%
Protein	25%
Fat	20%

We need to reaffirm that there is no magic fat-loss pill or tablet. If there were I would tell everyone and, let's face it, everyone would take it and the world wouldn't have a weight problem. If you're looking for one sure-fire method of weight loss that works for everyone, this is it. My clients and readers of *The Fat-Stripping Diet* have all been amazed at how they have lost fat and kept it off by following my eating plans.

Further compelling evidence can be found at the National Weight Control Registry (NWCR) in the United States. This organisation monitors people who have lost 13.6 kilograms or more and kept it off for over a year. Dr James Hill of the University of Colorado and Dr Rena Wing of the University of Pittsburgh started it in 1993. No supplements are being plugged here, nor are there any books, tapes or capsules, just real everyday people sharing their weight-loss strategies. There are thousands of people on this registry and their purpose is to tell you what they ate, how often they ate it and what else they did to achieve what everyone wants to achieve – weight loss.

Many of the group said that they had had enough of dieting through fad weight-loss measures such as food combining, high-protein no-carbohydrate diets or even high-fat diets. They were sick of looking at photos of themselves and feeling unhappy with what they saw. It turns out that the women ate only 35 grams of fat every day and the men consumed only 44 grams per day. This is well below the maximum levels of 41 and 60 grams respectively, which is what I have always advocated as the main aspect of fat loss. It also supports the fantastic results that people have achieved from following the 7×7 Fat-Reducing Plan.

In terms of how much real food this is during a typical day, these percentages translate to plenty of fruit, vegetables, brown breads, cereals and good-quality rice and pasta (the equivalent of two to two and a half small bowls of pasta a day) for carbohydrates; one piece of lean grilled steak, two glasses of milk and half a can of tuna for protein; and the equivalent of two glasses of low-fat high-calcium milk, a quarter of an avocado, one tablespoon of sunflower oil and two small scoops of low-fat ice cream for fat. As the breakdown of food shows, success comes from eating plenty of carbohydrates, which we will simply refer to as plant food.

Losing fat

To achieve permanent weight loss so that we look and feel our best, we have to reduce our fat intake. As we explained on pages 5–6, a woman's body will use 41 grams of fat each day. As the average woman eats 70 grams of fat, it means that she is eating 29 grams (70 – 41) too much. This excess fat results in the average woman needing to walk for 130 minutes a day just to metabolise this excess fat so that it does not get stored as body fat. Women simply do not have time to do this amount of exercise every day, so this 31 grams will get stored as fat. This fat storage could result in 11 kilograms of fat gained in a year! By reducing the amount of fat eaten each day to below 40 grams, the average woman would decrease the amount of energy she ate per day by roughly 17.5% or 1134 kJ per day. In seven days, this is about 8000 kJ, and a whopping 400 000 kJ per year. This would result in a huge fat loss – roughly 11 kilograms per year.

In Australia, the UK and the USA, a typical woman aged between twenty-five and forty-four eats 7800 kJ of energy each day. This is broken down into food groups accordingly (see page 19).

A man can consume 60 grams of fat each day with no fat being stored. However, the average man has 45 grams of excess fat (105–60). This means that the average bloke would need to walk about 100 minutes a day just to avoid storing fat. If he cut his fat to 60 grams then he would save 1701 kJ per day. Over seven days this is 11 907 kJ, and 620 000 kJ per year. This is enough to stay lean for life. However, this current excess of 46 grams per day is equivalent to 12–16 kilograms of fat gain in one year.

AVERAGE WOMAN'S DAILY INTAKE

FOOD GROUP	GRAMS	KILOJOULES	PERCENTAGE OF DAILY FOOD INTAKE
Carbohydrates	220	3696	47
Protein	76.2	1280	16
Fat	70	2646	34
Alcohol			3

The average man aged between twenty-five and forty-four eats 11 725 kJ of energy and his food is broken down in the following way.

AVERAGE MAN'S DAILY INTAKE

FOOD GROUP	GRAMS	KILOJOULES	PERCENTAGE OF DAILY FOOD INTAKE
Carbohydrates	316	5309	47
Protein	115.2	1932	16
Fat	105	3969	34
Alcohol			3

Understanding the simple processes involved in fat metabolism can empower you not only to reduce your body fat, but to live a longer and more energised life.

Fast fat loss

I want to share with you a story of a woman who lost massive amounts of weight on a high-protein diet. This woman lost 35 kilograms in about 15 weeks. Some people may think that's fantastic and cheer her on. But she lost this weight too quickly and lost muscle instead of fat. Her skin sagged. Her belly fell down just above her knees, and her skin hung underneath her arms. It looked as if she was wearing a jumper that was five sizes too big. She is typical of many who lose too much muscle and not fat. This is the wrong way to lose weight.

In summary

Fat loss must be viewed in the short, medium and long terms. With this outlook numerous people are keeping weight off and beating the yo-yo effect. Understanding how your body works, and how fads don't work is a very empowering and motivational tool for fat loss. Most importantly, you must understand that it is possible to lose weight.

FAT AND FOOD

Key messages for this chapter

YOU WILL DISCOVER:

- carbohydrates assist in weight loss
- high-protein diets are dangerous
- losing body fat has bonuses for your health
- how to reduce your body fat and live a longer, healthier life

How to eat

Guilt should not be a part of your eating habits. This chapter will help you to understand how food works in your body, so that you can take control of your eating plans. Rather than just being told to cut out chocolate or soft drinks without really knowing why, you'll choose to avoid those foods.

As discussed in Chapter 1, the female body will use about 41 grams of fat every day and the male body 60 grams. Eating more than this will lead to fat storage and eating less will lead to fat loss. This is a winning formula that has enabled many thousands of people to lose body fat and stay lean for many years. Not only is this a winning formula, it's also a simple formula. Put simply, if a woman eats 20 grams of fat for the day and her body needs 41 grams, then her body will use 21 grams (41 − 20) from her body-fat stores. If a man eats 25 grams of fat for the day, his body will use 35 grams (60 − 25) from his fat stores.

Understanding fat

Fats that come from animals, such as meat and dairy products, are called saturated fats. Saturated fats are used extensively in the fast food industry because they are very cheap. Burgers are usually fried in beef tallow, while doughnuts are immersed in thick emulsions of cooking lard. When you want to burn fat from your body, saturated fat is probably the hardest fat to remove. Animal fat goes into your fat cells first and is very hard to move due to its shape. Eating large amounts of saturated fat will lead to weight gain and in particular fat gain. On average people eat far too much animal fat: 25–36 grams a day for women and 40–55 grams a day for men. The problems that can result from increased weight include heart disease and diabetes, increased blood pressure and elevated cholesterol levels.

By following the 7×7 Fat-Reducing Plan, you will lose fat by reducing your fat intake, you will lose weight and keep it off. This is how you can be leaner and live longer. Very few eating plans can safely say that they can achieve this. So focus on following the eating plan in this book, and your stored fat will be used for energy and your body will be cleaned out, making it leaner and healthier.

Good fat

Fat contains a lot of energy – nearly two and a half times that of carbohydrates and proteins – but it isn't necessary to eliminate fat entirely from your diet. The body cannot produce the essential fats that are required for the nervous tissue, the eyes and brain; the production of hormones; blood clotting; muscle contraction; and control of blood pressure.

It makes sense that the eating plan you follow contains enough good fats but is low enough so that you don't store fat. In terms of good fat, all you need each day is one teaspoon of olive oil (mono-unsaturated fat) and one tablespoon of sunflower oil (polyunsaturated fat). One tablespoon of sunflower oil and one teaspoon of olive oil is about 17 grams. These fats eaten in small amounts will provide all the essential fats for your body and will not get converted to body fat.

Eating more than this will lead to you storing it as excess fat. It is still an area that people find confusing, but don't be tricked into thinking that because it's olive oil and good for cholesterol levels, it won't make you put on weight. Even too much good oil can make you fat. The next time you're watching your favorite cooking show and the chef uses lashings of olive oil, think hard before doing the same. Although good fats can reduce bad cholesterol levels and contain essential fatty acids, an excess can lead to long-term weight gain. This is a classic case of too much of a good thing.

If you ate 40 grams of fat a day for energy *plus* one tablespoon of sunflower oil and about a teaspoon of olive oil, could you can actually eat about 57 grams of fat a day without getting fat? The essential fats that we need in our diet do not get converted into body fat. So about 17 grams of essential fats from about a tablespoon of sunflower oil and about a teaspoon of olive oil will be used for other roles in the body. This means you still have 40 grams maximum to eat during the day. In this case, you could eat 57 grams of fat for the day and still not store fat. The challenge for you is to get your 17 grams of good fats within your 40 gram fat allowance.

Many people think that you need fat for energy, which is true, but they use it as an excuse to eat lots of fat. The fact is that we have enough fat on our bodies to last a very long time.

People who get lost in the desert or the bush are able to survive many days without eating just because of their fat stores.

Understanding carbohydrates

Carbohydrates are produced from the most natural ingredients found on earth – water, carbon dioxide, and sunlight. This simple yet incredibly effective cocktail of nature is combined in plants. When plants are cultivated and the heads of, say, wheat are crushed and soaked, then boiled, an edible carbohydrate is formed. Carbohydrates such as rice, maize, corn, and cassava have been a staple part of many cultures' diets for centuries. All carbohydrates are broken down into a useable form in the body called glucose. This glucose is stored as glycogen in the liver and muscle cells. When plant material is processed in the body further, sugar (glucose) is produced. Sugar is a simple carbohydrate, which is broken down quickly to glucose and used as energy in the body. Complex carbohydrates, such as bread, rice, pasta and cereals, are broken down more slowly.

Today complex carbohydrates are readily available; bread, cereals, grains, pastas, rice, corn, fruit and most vegetables fall into this category. People tend to forget when they talk about carbohydrates that fruit and most vegetables are predominantly part of this food group. The notion of eliminating carbohydrates from any diet seems almost impossible, impractical and unsafe.

Carbohydrates perform many primary and secondary functions in the body. The primary function is to maintain a continuous supply of glucose to the brain and nervous system. Each day the brain needs 120–180 grams of glucose to carry out its billion simultaneous functions, such as thinking, processing information, muscle contraction and keeping the heart beating. Some people have called this requirement 'carbohydrate cravings', and deemed it a bad thing. However, the natural functioning of our brain requires glucose. People who don't eat carbohydrates are unable to concentrate for long periods of time. If you ever try to concentrate or work while hungry, you will find that you don't have the ability to focus because your brain doesn't have the energy to function properly. This is because your brain is using more glucose than usual, and hence more energy. Recent evidence also shows that an adequate supply of glucose is required by the heart muscle.

Carbohydrates are stored as glycogen in the liver and muscle cells, which can hold 70 grams and 400 grams respectively. In Western societies these stores are never completely full, because we eat so much fat and relatively little carbohydrate in comparison. Carbohydrates also have a hydrating effect on the body, because every gram of glycogen (stored glucose) is bound to 3–4 grams of water. Hydration is essential for the human body, and most people are aware that they need to drink plenty of water. But have you ever wondered where water is primarily stored? If your carbohydrate intake is low, you will often feel thirsty and dehydrated. Your glycogen stores will be low, which in turn means that water has nothing to bind itself to.

Carbohydrates are important

Carbohydrates together with fat are responsible for the supply of energy for the reactions that take place in the body. Thousands of small yet significant metabolic reactions take place in the body every day. Your body burns large amounts of energy when you sleep because that's when your metabolism works hard to break down, digest and store food nutrients, and to keep the body breathing. Your brain still thinks and processes information, and of course your body is continually repairing cells, and producing enzymes and hormones.

The simple process of replacing fat with plant-based carbohydrates will reduce body fat. If you recall the National Weight Control Registry in the USA clearly demonstrates that when you consume nearly two-thirds of your food from plant food, then fat loss can continue for as long as you follow this eating plan (see Chapter 3). Imagine losing an average of 30 kilograms and keeping it off for years. This doesn't mean that everyone has 30 kilograms to lose, though. Even if it's just 3 or 4 kilograms, then the 7×7 Fat-Reducing Plan is still incredibly effective. This is also a plan that you can stick to in the long term. If it's body fat you want to lose in both the short and long term, then you cannot go past carbohydrates such as cereals and grains (including rice, pasta, wholemeal bread and muesli), fruits and vegetables (including bananas, potatoes and pumpkins) and legumes (including lentils, chickpeas and kidney beans). This doesn't mean that we have to overeat these foods. Of course you shouldn't eat four or five large bowls of pasta or ten potatoes a day, but you should make these your base foods.

In countries where complex carbohydrates are traditionally the staple food, body fat is at a minimum. The further benefits from eating complex carbohydrates are numerous and include a marked reduction in cholesterol levels and a decreased risk of colon cancer. Weight control and weight loss through the consumption of complex carbohydrates has been the cornerstone of success at B Personal.

Is sugar a carbohydrate?

Complex carbohydrates are beneficial because they are low in fat, they protect our heart from disease, protect us from certain cancers, and provide vitamins, minerals and balance to our health. We need to eat carbohydrates that are less processed, which includes cereals, brown bread, potatoes and rice. And we do eat too many sweets and drink too many soft drinks. Our children are the worst offenders in this case.

Many people confuse sugar and chocolate. Chocolate is very high in fat. But chocolate is sugary and fattening, isn't it? Six squares of chocolate contain 624 kJ of energy. They also contain 7.9 grams of fat (the milk fats that give chocolate a solid look and smooth mouth feel) and 18 grams of sugar. There is 300 kJ of energy from chocolate (48% fat), and 133 kJ of energy from sugar (21% sugar). As we know, the sugar is converted and stored as glycogen. However, the fat in chocolate is stored as fat. To walk off a chocolate bar can take about 100 minutes, between

8 and 10 kilometres. A slice of cheesecake has 1400 kJ of energy: 22 grams of fat (831 kJ at 60% fat) and 29.5 grams of sugar (496 kJ at 35% sugar). In these cases it is not the sugar that is fattening but rather the large amounts of fat. The sugar will be converted to glycogen and stored in about one hour.

Doctors and nutritionists advise people not to eat so much sugar. The reason for this is *not* because they think that sugar will make you fat, but because sugar is energy that takes the room of more important, more valuable foods that the body needs. Eating too many sugary foods such as soft drinks, lollies and confectionery takes up room in our diet, allowing little room for fruit, vegetables and fibre and water.

CUT DOWN ON SUGAR

We need to cut down on sugar because it contains 'empty calories'. Although sugar doesn't convert to fat, the energy (glucose) from sugar contains no vitamins, minerals, or fibre. To date there is absolutely no medical evidence that sugar gets converted to fat.

The detoxing myth

So many people go on detoxing diets for various reasons, believing that they can cleanse their bodies of 'toxins' by restricting all forms of carbohydrates. By eating less sugar and drinking less alcohol while consuming more nutritious foods, you will feel better, and undoubtedly you'll have more energy.

You don't need a brain surgeon to tell you that. Flushing out toxins, aiding weight loss, and getting rid of the toxins that cause cellulite are some of the extravagant claims made by advocates of 'detoxing'. Still the most common question I hear is how do I get rid of cellulite? Toxins or waste do not cause it, and there are no tablets, creams or deep tissue massage that can get rid of it. Cellulite is fat that is held in place by connective tissue. The more fat you eat, the more fat you will store. As you will see later, you need to empty your fat cells by a combination of factors, not by cutting out carbohydrates to detoxify your body. Anything toxic in your body that hangs around long enough will seriously harm you. This is why the liver does all the removal of any harmful substance for you. Folks, you cannot detox your body!

Protein

Protein is a linkage of smaller molecules called amino acids, which are found abundantly in plant materials and in meat and fish. Amino acids are involved in many functions throughout the human body. The greatest function is the passing of genetic material on to form new cells in the brain, nerves, eyes, ears, heart muscles and respiratory organs, to name just a few. The formation of new cells is essential to our survival and growth.

Protein is also involved in the production of hormones such as insulin, adrenaline and seratonin, and sex hormones; the production of vital enzymes, including those that break down foods in your stomach; and making transport proteins, which deliver molecules from the intestine to specific parts of the body or from one part of the body to another. For example, haemoglobin, a transport protein, is the chief molecule that takes oxygen from the lungs to the cells of the body. Protein is also needed for the healthy growth of hair and nails, connective tissue such as elastin and collagen, and making immune-system antibodies. In the immune system there are around eleven proteins that work together. Proteins also help muscle tissue growth and repair.

The metabolism (digestion, absorption and storage) of large amounts of protein is very slow. The body cannot break down protein quickly. Even the most rapidly digestible protein – whey protein – is absorbed at only 6–7 grams per hour. When protein is broken down it releases amino acids into the bloodstream. These amino acids release glucose and insulin, which in turn drives the amino acids into liver and muscle tissue where they can be used for the necessary functions. Protein cannot be stored in the body. Therefore it is continuously being recycled in the body's 'protein pool'. Because of their functional diversity, proteins can be broken down and reassembled by the human body, depending on the requirement at the time.

About 300 grams of protein is broken down and reconstructed every day. This means that the recycling of enzymes, free amino acids, muscle proteins and hormones is essential to produce the most necessary protein on a daily basis. After weight training or muscle injury, for example, muscle repair is essential. After surgery, proteins responsible for making haemoglobin take precedence over other protein needs. There may be a need to increase protein intake for the elderly, and also for those who are active. Once these needs are met, protein is broken down and urinated out as urea.

Be careful of including too many processed proteins in your diet. We know growth hormones, steroids and antibiotics, and colourings are primary examples of the additives in many processed proteins. How this effects our bodies long-term is still under review, but we do know that the antibiotics fed to cattle, for example, are making bacteria immune to the antibiotics, allowing them to multiply and spread rapidly. We know also that there is a strong association between red meat consumption and cancer, although we are not sure exactly why. In Western societies the amount of protein we eat (especially meat) has increased rapidly in the last ten years.

People also tend to replace carbohydrates with large amounts of fat so, as you are now well aware, eating fat will lead to fat storage. However, the high intake of animal protein produces chemicals in our bodies that not too many people are aware of. Animal proteins contain amino acids that are rich in sulphur. These sulphur-rich amino acids don't quite break down fully and produce a substance called homocysteine. This substance is considered very dangerous and leads to heart disease.

Eating large amounts of protein may actually fill you up more than fat or carbohydrates, causing you to eat less, which means you might not have the necessary intake of fibre and energy. As the chart on page 37 shows, there are many more complications from eating large amounts of protein, especially at the expense of plant food.

High carbohydrates vs high protein

Undoubtedly one of the great scientific debates that rages today is that between carbohydrates and protein. Both are essential for growth of the human body, but people have been advised to go to extremes. Some people eliminate all carbohydrates from their diet while others eliminate all proteins. And high-protein, low-carbohydrate diets are among the most popular today. I'm amazed at how many people are willing to give up some of the most important (and low-fat) foods – bread, pasta, rice – in their quest to lose weight.

Moderate amounts of protein are essential for our bodies and moderate consumption helps to make you feel full after a meal. Carbohydrates provide the energy we need for our metabolisms to work effectively and to go about our daily lives. There is no point having all the equipment (protein) for growth but no energy (carbohydrate) to carry out the repairs. Carbohydrates are the only energy source for the brain and nervous system (see page 26). Do we dare deprive the most important organ in the human body – the brain – of its fuel?

The carbohydrate myth

The myth about sugar or carbohydrates being converted into fat (bread, rice, potatoes, bananas, pasta and sugar turning to fat) is one of the biggest 'cons' of the twenty-first century. Remember that any carbohydrate will be converted to glucose, not fat, and then stored as glycogen in muscle and liver cells. How is it then that many people are concerned that a potato or a bowl of rice will be converted into fat?

ONLY FAT IS STORED AS FAT

30 grams of jelly babies would be converted to and stored as glycogen. It would never be converted to fat, so you don't have to walk it off.

30 grams of fat from cheese would be converted to fat. It would take 95 minutes, about 10 kilometres, to walk off.

Recent studies show that single meals containing as much as 500–700 grams of carbohydrate (equivalent of 1500 grams of cooked pasta) produced no fat storage, but rather glycogen storage. If you consider that the average bowl of rice or pasta contains 50–75 grams of carbohydrate, then even if normal semi-active people consumed eight large bowls of pasta in a single day they would still not store fat. But realistically how many people would eat this much food anyway?

Other studies of massive overfeeding of 1500 grams of carbohydrate in the form of pasta showed that after two and a half days the carbohydrate (glucose) still converted to glycogen not fat. From these studies and numerous others it is known that 700–1000 grams of carbohydrate can be effectively used by the body each day as glycogen, not fat.

> The average man eats 300 grams of carbohydrates per day. The average woman eats 210 grams.

In the seventies and eighties, the theory of converting carbohydrates to fat seemed feasible, due to lack of finely researched science. At that time, computers were the size of telephone booths, mobile phones were not in circulation, the Internet was a mere theory, and cloning was science fiction. With the giant leaps of science, technology and equipment, we can now see the biochemical pathways of what happens when sugar or carbohydrates are eaten. We are now able to see and photograph carbohydrates being stored as glycogen. They look like tiny clusters of pepper joined together in a star-like formation. Whether we eat one potato or ten, the body does not convert them into fat but glycogen. This process is the quickest in the body and takes about one hour.

When you eat more plant food than fat, there are several advantages. Your body uses more energy to break down carbohydrates and store it as glycogen. This uses three times more energy than it does to store fat. Storing fat takes hardly any energy. If you are eating mainly carbohydrates, then your fat intake is reduced and so no fat will be stored. But your body still needs to use fat, which will come from your fat stores or excess body fat. This is how you lose fat and weight.

We never overeat on carbohydrates but on fat. We know that excess carbohydrates are stored as glycogen and used rapidly as fuel for the body's processes. What about excess fat? This is our main concern. For reactions requiring quick bursts of energy, such as running for the train, that energy is supplied by glucose. For ongoing reactions, such as digestion and the transport of nutrients around the body, slower energy pathways may be used, supplied by fat.

High-protein diets

If you stay on a high-protein diet for any length of time, you are likely to experience one or more of the following problems:

- loss of muscle, because the body needs to convert amino acids (muscle) into glucose for the brain and nervous system
- low levels of stored glucose (glycogen), hence the breaking down of muscle
- headaches and migraines, from dehydration. Water binds to glycogen (from carbohydrates) to keep you hydrated (see page 26).

Clients who have previously been on high-protein diets tell me that they drink plenty of water but are always thirsty. Small stores of carbohydrates mean small stores of glycogen and water. The water passes straight through you rather than being

THE RISKS AND REALITIES OF HIGH-PROTEIN DIETS

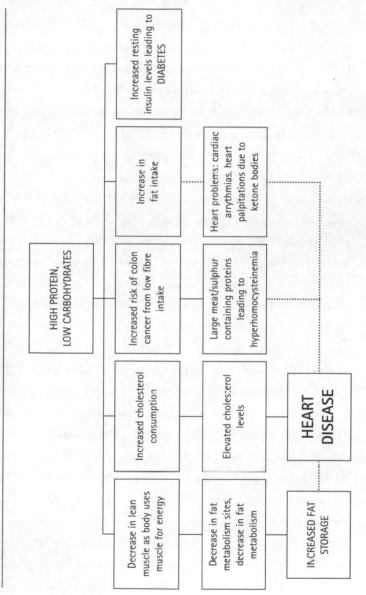

held in the body. This can lead to long-term deficiencies in water-soluble vitamins such as vitamin C and most vitamin Bs. If fat is burnt or used up in muscle cells and you are losing muscle, it simply means you will burn less fat.

Many of my clients have been on a high-protein and low-carbohydrate diet. This is a diet focused on eating plenty of red meat, chicken, fish, eggs and protein supplements. In some cases only small amounts of vegetables are eaten. No rice, pasta, bread or cereals are allowed. It's true that some people will have some short-term weight loss, after about five or six weeks. Scientists have questioned whether it is the high-protein intake that brings about this weight loss or simply the lack of food that people endure when on a high-protein diet. Studies have found that people who follow high-protein diets eat about 2100 kJ less each day than people following a normal eating regime. Consuming such low amounts of food qualifies as food restriction, which is why people cannot sustain these diets for long periods of time.

Interestingly, people who have restricted their intake by 2100 kJ but continued to eat carbohydrates found that there was no difference in the amount of weight lost. The weight loss comes from a low intake of calories, not from eliminating carbohydrates. However, when carbohydrates were included in the diet there was less muscle loss and more actual fat loss. High-protein diets don't actually help you to lose weight any more significantly than a high-percentage carbohydrate diet.

It is very hard to eat a high-protein diet for long periods of time because of continual tiredness, lethargy, lack of energy and constipation. However, it is very common for people with no study in the area of nutrition or metabolism to advocate high-protein diets. As mounting evidence suggests, eating large amounts of protein can have very serious and dangerous side effects. Although the most common side effects are bad breath, lack of concentration and kidney damage, some not so commonly known are:

- heart arrhythmia
- wasting of valuable heart muscle
- decreases in heart contraction
- osteoporosis
- cancer (from increased red meat intake)
- the breakdown of cardiac muscle (heart muscle), to be used for energy when carbohydrates are scarce
- sudden death

'As long as I lose weight, I don't care about anything else.' I've heard many people claim that they don't care if their health suffers, as long as they can be thin. Although they may be aware of the adverse side effects of high-protein diets, some people cannot be deterred from eating copious amounts of protein. This chapter is important for all those following high-protein diets without regard to the potential damage. Recent studies of the nutritional value of low-carbohydrate diets show that they are deficient in fibre, thiamin, folate, vitamins A, E and B_6, calcium, magnesium, iron and potassium.

High-protein diets produce an excess of ketone bodies. These are the leftover products from using protein and fat for energy when there are no carbohydrates available. These ketone bodies make the blood more acidic and decrease its ability to carry oxygen. They also put a strain on the kidneys, which have to work harder to filter them out. Ketone bodies drag other important particles such as sodium, potassium and calcium away from the blood. These three elements are responsible for keeping the heartbeat constant, and disruption to them can lead to serious health implications.

How it all works

During the day a person can eat only so much. If your diet consists of, say, 60–70 per cent protein, then you could be eating between 200 grams (women) and 300 grams (men) of protein per day. There are a few points to consider here. First, eating foods such as red meat, chicken, fish, eggs and protein supplements amounts to a very expensive shopping list. Secondly, meats such as beef and lamb contain cholesterol. This high-protein intake could potentially amount to 750–1100 mg of cholesterol per day. Several of my clients were eating eight to ten eggs per day just to keep up their protein. This corresponds to 2000 mg of cholesterol per day in the eggs alone. The body alone produces 1000 mg of cholesterol each day. Although individual serves of food might be low in cholesterol, their total sum for the day could be very large. The recommended cholesterol intake is 300 mg per day.

Thirdly, there are limited amounts of fruit and vegetables in a high-protein diet. High-protein advocates still fail to call fruit and vegetables 'carbohydrates'. Fruits and vegetables are needed for their vitamin, mineral and essential fatty acid contents, but also equally importantly because of their fibre content. Fibre is the skin or part of the fruit or vegetable that remains partly undigested and passes through the body very quickly. In doing so it can make you feel full, because it absorbs water and fills you up, but also takes digested food particles with it. This means that any potential carcinogenic particle, from processed foods, for example, that is sitting in your intestine has no time to react. It is dragged out with the fibre. Remember, colon cancer is the third most common cancer worldwide, and a lack of fruit and vegetables in your diet will increase your risk of developing it. I am stunned when clients come to me after being on a high-protein diet for several weeks. Some don't go to the toilet for five days straight. When I analyse their diets, it is very obvious that their intake of fruit and vegetables is very low. Apart from fibre, there are other non-nutritive components in fruit and vegetables that are reported to be beneficial in reducing the risk of cancer.

Some people feel that they become bloated when they eat carbohydrates. It's true that some people develop an inability to digest carbohydrates derived from wheat. This condition is called gluten intolerance or coeliac disease. If you do experience problems with bloating, you can be allergy-tested to see if that is what is causing the discomfort. Even if you are gluten-intolerant, you can still eat rice and corn-based pastas without any problems. Coeliac disease is hereditary, and is not caused by eating too much pasta. Women twenty-five years old and above are particularly prone to this gluten intolerance.

Carbohydrates and insulin

One of the most forceful arguments that high-protein advocates use is that carbohydrates raise insulin levels, and therefore fat storage is increased when a diet includes carbohydrates. Whenever you eat carbohydrates, they are broken down into small glucose pieces. These glucose pieces need to be transported to muscle and liver cells where they can be stored. Like a taxi, insulin (which is made in the pancreas) transports glucose to the muscle and liver cells where this energy source can be called upon by the brain and nervous system at a later stage.

After you eat a meal, the blood contains increased levels of glucose, amino acids (from protein) and fat. These nutrients need to be cleared away from the bloodstream and used by the body. Insulin helps move these nutrients into storage sites and stops them from being leaked back into the bloodstream. For example, while storing glucose in the liver, insulin also prevents glucose that is already in the liver from being released.

Insulin levels rise in the bloodstream primarily to restore balance to the blood. The rise in insulin occurs roughly ten to

INSULIN RESPONSE TO CARBOHYDRATES

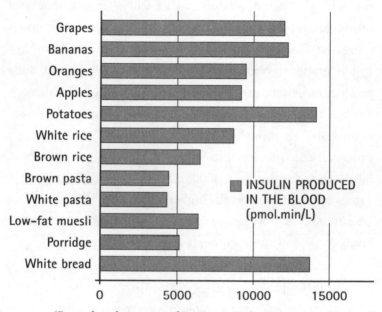

(Reproduced courtesy of Dr Susan Holt, University of Sydney)

twelve minutes after you eat. There are two bursts of insulin after a meal, a quick burst and a second slow, prolonged burst. Levels subside about two hours after a big meal. After a small snack insulin levels in the blood fall much faster (after about 20 minutes).

This is where the high-protein argument becomes unstuck, because whenever you eat a meal insulin will always be produced. Insulin is a very misunderstood hormone and due to this misunderstanding it has been touted as the reason people get fat. Many people say that if you eat foods that raise insulin, you will get fat. The reason is that when large amounts of insulin are present in your bloodstream after a meal, fat use is decreased. However, proteins *and* carbohydrates raise insulin.

The graph on page 43 shows how much insulin our body produces when we eat carbohydrates. Complex carbohydrates such as pasta, porridge, muesli and rice raise insulin levels comparable to those obtained from eating fish, which is a protein (see page 46). Brown pasta raises insulin to about 5000, white rice to about 8000, and potatoes to about 14 000. Fruits raise insulin levels higher than complex pastas do because they are broken down much faster. However, insulin levels come down more quickly after eating fruit.

INSULIN: is it about weight?

The brain functions on glucose and glucose alone. Without adequate glucose travelling to the brain, a person becomes jittery, lacks concentration, makes simple basic errors or faints. Normally we run low on glucose at about 10.30 a.m. and 3 p.m. This is called hypoglycaemia or low blood sugar. In order for glucose to get to the brain, a hormone called insulin pushes it. Insulin is produced continuously by the pancreas during a normal twenty-four hour period and keeps glucose travelling to the brain constantly. For this reason insulin is *always* present in our bloodstream at low levels (50–120 pm).

Protein and insulin

Why does protein raise insulin? Protein is broken down into amino acids and absorbed into the bloodstream from our intestine. These amino acids partly break down into glucose themselves (a process called gluconeogenesis) and/or signal to the liver to release glucose into the blood. This results in a barrage of insulin being released. This insulin is needed not only to pack carbohydrates (glucose) into muscle cells and fat into fat cells, but also to transport amino acids into muscle and liver cells. Hence insulin provides the bus ride that amino acids need to get from the intestine, through the blood to muscle and liver cells for further processing.

Using advanced measurement techniques, we now know that the major fate of protein in our diet is conversion into glucose. It has been shown that for every 100 grams of protein eaten, 50–60 per cent is converted into glucose.

As the chart on page 46 shows, protein-containing foods dramatically raise insulin. Baked beans produce an insulin response of over 20 000, which is well above the resting insulin level of 50 to 120. Fish, lentils and beef all produce comparable if not increased levels of insulin when compared with some carbohydrates.

Insulin is always present in the blood. Fish and lentils raise insulin to 9200–9350 which is over ninety times resting levels, followed by beef, 80 times resting levels, cheese and eggs which raise insulin 47 and 60 times respectively. The only difference when protein raises insulin is that because protein metabolism

INSULIN RESPONSE TO PROTEIN

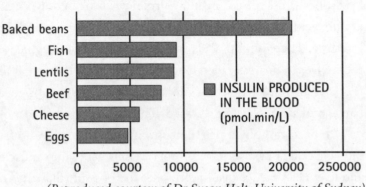

(Reproduced courtesy of Dr Susan Holt, University of Sydney)

is slow, protein raises insulin and keeps it raised for eight to ten hours after you have finished eating. Carbohydrates raise insulin but these levels drop in about one hour. As you can see, the effects of protein on raising insulin and keeping it raised can be dangerous.

SCIENTIFIC BREAKTHROUGHS

While many people are still focused on the fad-diet insulin theory, scientists have moved forward into new areas of research. The hormone in the spotlight at the moment is leptin, a chemical produced by fat cells that works in partnership with insulin, telling the brain to store fat, use fat and even destroy fat cells. Some preliminary studies show that when leptin is injected into mice, body fat drops by 78 per cent, despite elevated insulin levels.

Remember that the anti-carbohydrate scientists tell us to eliminate carbohydrates specifically because they raise insulin. This graph is important for you to understand completely that all foods raise insulin. In the quest to lose weight, many people focus on trying to balance insulin in the belief that raising insulin levels will make them fat. But as you can see, whenever you eat and whatever you eat, insulin levels are raised. People trying to balance their insulin levels are focused on the wrong aspect of weight loss.

Weight loss is about reducing your fat intake. Nothing more, nothing less.

Eating carbohydrates late in the day

Cutting down on carbohydrates after lunch or after 6 p.m. has no scientific basis. Carbohydrates are converted to glycogen (not fat) at any time of the day. We need to eat less fat rather than less carbohydrate. In fact, we actually need to reduce our total food intake. We all tend to eat too much food, eating until we're full at every meal. This is our downfall.

People who don't eat carbohydrates after midday or 6 p.m. run the risk of consuming low amounts of fibre and energy. Even eating non-starchy vegetables would only give them 3 grams of fibre. This means they would need to consume 27 grams of fibre before midday, which is very impractical (two bananas, two apples, a pear and four Weet-Bix). There is strong evidence to suggest that the 'no carbs after lunch' rule falls into the low-carbohydrate category, with all the health risks that entails.

Permanent fat loss

Eating a high percentage of carbohydrates can make you lose fat weight. However, this book does not advocate overeating carbohydrates or any other food group. Balanced eating with a high percentage of carbohydrates is the foundation for permanent fat loss. Eating less fat than 41 grams for women and 60 grams for men means that the body will take fat from your body to use as energy. You might ask what would happen if you ate high protein and low fat. Unfortunately you would lose precious muscle cells for energy. This is because protein metabolism is slow. To make glucose in the absence of carbohydrates the body goes first to its muscle stores (including heart muscle), not its fat stores. You cannot speed up fat metabolism by cutting out carbohydrates, so you will lose valuable muscle and water and retain fat. That's why you may lose weight but retain cellulite. When you go off a protein diet, you will store more fat because by losing lean muscle you have lost fat-burning sites. The less muscle you have on your body, the slower your metabolism. The more muscle, the higher your metabolic rate.

In summary

By consuming predominantly carbohydrates, you will retain muscle and lose fat weight. Continue along this path long-term and you will keep fat off for good. Eating sensible amounts of carbohydrates will give you enough energy for all your daily needs without letting you store fat.

CHAPTER 3

THE 7×7
FAT-REDUCING
PLAN

Key messages for this chapter

YOU WILL DISCOVER:

- how to eat all the time without overeating
- that weight loss doesn't happen through deprivation
- that the 7×7 Fat-Reducing Plan works best when you are prepared
- the seven successful strategies to strip fat

The seven-day plan

Seven meals a day seems like a mighty tall ask, you may think, but it is the way forward in effective fat stripping. Cultures that exhibit very good health as well as good weight control don't gorge or eat to full capacity. The emphasis is on grazing. These concepts may seem tough for a bloke who loves to go to the 'all you can eat' restaurant, but this chapter will put things in perspective. Having spent over a year living in Italy, I found that eating several small meals a day is normal. You may even have four courses in one meal but they are small serves, as in this plan.

The problem with only three meals a day is that people just love to eat. We eat without really thinking about it. These three meals tend to be large but then we usually sneak some junk food in between as well. The aim of the 7×7 Fat-Reducing Plan is to:

- eat less food more often, so as not to overeat or eat in between meals
- keep fat intake down
- increase fibre intake
- reduce the amount of energy we eat
- consume enough nutrients
- lose body fat.

The focus of the eating plan is, like the very successful Fat-Stripping Diet, to keep fat intake to a minimum, thus allowing your body to use its own fat stores for energy, and to increase fibre intake. This book takes the concept further. It breaks your food into much smaller meals and speeds up your metabolism. The faster you burn this food up, the faster your metabolism and the faster you burn fat. One of the keys to success with this eating plan is to include vegetables or salad with every evening meal. You must eat these first and finish them before you eat the rest of your meal.

Fibre and energy density

People need to reduce the amount of sugar they eat to make room for more fibre. Although the amount of fibre consumed by Australian adults is reported to be over 20 grams per day (it is recommended we eat over 30 grams), many health professionals suggest that this value is actually much less. In the United States some reports show the average American struggles to consume 15 grams of fibre each day, opting more for a no-fibre fast food burger and fries.

So why is substituting fat for fibre a more healthful choice than fat for low fat? Fibre-containing foods are much more filling than low-fibre food. For example, eating two bananas is much more filling than eating a fast food burger. The banana contains 3 grams of fibre, no fat, 1000 kJ of energy and will fill you up. A fast food burger and ice cream contains 0.2 grams of fibre, 42 grams of fat, 4000 kJ of energy. Studies show the lack of fibre and large amount of fat in such a meal will leave you hungry only a few hours later. The energy density of the fast food option is four times as great as the high-fibre banana option.

Deprivation is not the answer

Depriving yourself of food you love is not the answer to successful short- and long-term fat loss. It is certainly not part of the 7×7 Fat-Reducing Plan. Can you honestly stay on a diet that says you can't eat chocolate? I have asked thousands of men and women if they would cheat and eat chocolate even if they were on a very strict diet. Most of them (99 per cent) say they have done so and would do so again. This is human nature.

I'll show you that you don't have to compromise your chocolate cravings just to keep fat off your body. Within the structure of the 7×7 Fat-Reducing Plan, your fat intake is low but it contains enough good fats to meet the body's needs.

THE 7×7 FAT-REDUCING PLAN

MONDAY	
mealtime	food
breakfast	1 high-fibre muffin, with a scraping of margarine & vegemite
	1 glass of orange juice
mid-morning snack	1 banana
	1 orange or other fruit
lunch	½–1 pita bread with salad & ham
	2 glasses of water
mid-afternoon snack	1 small tub of low-fat yoghurt
late-afternoon snack	1 apple

mealtime	food
dinner	large bowl of homemade vegetable soup with 2 pieces of bread
	1 glass of water
dessert	fresh fruit salad

▶ TUESDAY

mealtime	food
breakfast	small bowl of oats, with low-fat milk
	1 glass of orange juice
mid-morning snack	1 banana
	1 orange or other fruit
lunch	bowl of spicy broth with 1–2 pieces of bread
	2 glasses of water
mid-afternoon snack	1 slice of fruit bread
late-afternoon snack	1 small tub of low-fat yoghurt
	1 mandarin
dinner	2 servings of legumes such as chickpeas and lentils, with rice
	1 glass of water
dessert	1 small scoop of low-fat ice cream

▶ WEDNESDAY

mealtime	food
breakfast	2 pieces of fruit bread, with a scraping of margarine & strawberry jam
	1 glass of orange juice

mealtime	food
mid-morning snack	1 banana
	1 orange or other fruit
lunch	low-fat Caesar salad with 1–2 pieces of bread
	2 glasses of water
mid-afternoon snack	1 pear or other fruit option
late-afternoon snack	1 muesli bar
dinner	1 small bowl of pasta with seafood or lean lamb sauce, with salad
	1 glass of water
dessert	fresh fruit platter

▶ **THURSDAY**

mealtime	food
breakfast	small bowl of low-fat cereal, with low-fat milk & fruit
	1 glass of orange juice
mid-morning snack	1 banana
	1 orange or other fruit
lunch	½–1 salmon and salad sandwich or roll
	2 glasses of water
mid-afternoon snack	1 muesli bar
late-afternoon snack	1 small tub of low-fat yoghurt
dinner	a small piece of lean beef, & 2 different servings of legumes, with vegetables & rice
	1 glass of water
dessert	1 small scoop of gelati

▶ FRIDAY	
mealtime	**food**
breakfast	2 pieces of wholemeal toast, with a scraping of margarine & jam
	1 glass of orange juice
mid-morning snack	1 banana
	1 orange or other fruit
lunch	½–1 pita bread with roast beef & salad
	2 glasses of water
mid-afternoon snack	1 apple or other fruit
late-afternoon snack	1 muesli bar
dinner	grilled or baked fish or chicken with steamed vegetables or a small bowl of pasta with a tomato-based sauce & salad
	1 glass of red wine
dessert	fresh fruit platter

▶ SATURDAY	
mealtime	**food**
breakfast	banana smoothie, with low-fat milk
mid-morning snack	1 banana
	1 orange or other fruit
lunch	½–1 tuna and salad sandwich or roll
	2 glasses of water
mid-afternoon snack	4–5 rice crackers with low-fat tzatziki dip
late-afternoon snack	1 small tub of low-fat yoghurt
	1 orange

mealtime	food
dinner	grilled or baked fish with steamed
	vegetables, or a small bowl of pasta
	with a tomato-based sauce & salad
	1 glass of red wine & 1 glass of water
dessert	1 small scoop of low-fat frozen yoghurt

▶ **SUNDAY**

mealtime	food
breakfast	2 Weet-Bix, with low-fat milk
	1 glass of orange juice
mid-morning snack	1 banana
	1 orange or other fruit
lunch	your choice
mid-afternoon snack	1 small tub of low-fat yoghurt
late-afternoon snack	1 muesli bar
	1 apple
dinner	your choice
dessert	your choice

As you can see, these are not seven large meals that have you bursting at the seams, nor are there complicated ratios of foods that require hours to prepare. They are seven opportunities to eat during the day.

Fish has been included regularly on the menu, but if you dislike fish take some fish oil supplements every two or three days. Remember this fish oil in recommended amounts doesn't get converted to fat but rather hormones that are involved in regulating your blood pressure. The 7×7 Fat-Reducing Plan includes a variety of legumes such as chickpeas, red kidney beans and lentils. These foods promote healthy fat loss. It's important to try to include some in this eating plan once or twice a week. Include a vegetable soup, with plenty of different coloured vegetables, at least once or twice a week.

OFF THE MENU

- cheese, butter or cream, including creamy soups or pasta sauces
- full-cream milk (use low-fat milk that is high in calcium)
- full-fat yoghurt or ice cream
- coconut cream/milk dishes
- chicken with skin
- bacon with rind
- meat with fat on it (use only lean meats, including lean mince)
- fast food
- potato cakes, dim sims or other deep-fried food
- peanut butter (one tablespoon contains about 13 grams of fat)

Each meal is quite small, but if you feel full after breakfast, lunch or dinner, reduce the amount you are eating each time because another meal is around the corner. For example, if you have eaten breakfast and your mid-morning snack, and find that half a stuffed pita bread is too much, then you can either cut down your mid-morning snack to, say, half a banana and half an orange, or cut down your lunch to a quarter to half a pita bread.

BREAKFAST TIPS

- never skip breakfast
- always use low-fat high-calcium milk
- use only low-fat yoghurt
- fruit on its own for breakfast is a no-no, except for bananas
- if you struggle to eat breakfast, drink it in the form of a banana smoothie or Sustagen
- coffee and tea are fine (maximum 2–3 cups per day), but if you add sugar, keep it down to ½ to 1 teaspoon per cup
- eating breakfast on the go is fine: muesli bars are great in this instance

Alternatively, if you find that you are hungry after lunch, then eat a larger mid-morning snack next time around, rather than more lunch. For example, for your mid-morning snack eat two bananas, an apple and one stuffed pita bread, rather than two stuffed pita breads. Men in particular may find that they need to bolster their mid-morning snack, as they generally eat more than women do. If you are still hungry by mid-afternoon, you may need to adjust the amount of food you eat at lunch. Increase your lunch portion slightly or increase the food intake for your mid- or late-afternoon snack. This may take some trial and error but get it sorted out early in the program. If during a meal you are tempted to eat more out of sheer habit, you must try to resist. Wait ten minutes and you'll probably realise that you do feel full. Whenever possible, drink one or two glasses of water with all your meals. Water keeps you hydrated and you'll feel better with regular consumption.

The aim of this book is to remove the focus from the traditional three main meals: breakfast, lunch and dinner. Eating between meals is important, and the emphasis should be on maintaining your energy levels consistently throughout the day, with regular snacks.

The other feature of this eating plan is its flexibility. I've recommended seven meals for seven days and you can interchange Monday's lunch for Thursday's and so on. It's important to adhere to the number of meals for each day, but within the plan you can choose from each of the seven different breakfasts, snacks, lunches, dinners and desserts. It's a great idea to photocopy the plan and stick it on your fridge. Then whenever you are hungry, you can go the fridge and check what's available and what's allowed.

Danger time

The time between lunch and dinner is when many people get extremely hungry. This is also the most likely time for people following an eating plan to slip up. That's why there are two snack breaks here. Now you may not need to use the first one, which is fine. Just don't use it. There's no point eating when you are not hungry, but it is there because some people do get famished between lunch and dinner. So often, this is the time when you may be tempted to buy a potato cake, dim sims or even a hamburger before you get on the train home after work. It may even be a packet of salt and vinegar chips and a can of soft drink that fill the void. But all they really do is fill you up with fat, deprive you of fibre and reinforce the need to be prepared. Following the 7×7 Fat-Reducing Plan doesn't work if you don't have food with you at these times. Get into good habits early and be prepared. Once again take note that these small snacks are just that: small snacks, not overwhelming meals.

DINNER ALTERNATIVES

- tomato bruschetta
- lentil, chickpea and red kidney bean soup
- lentil and vegetable soup with two pieces of bread
- homemade Vietnamese rice paper rolls
- homemade sushi/nori rolls
- chicken pasta with legume salad
- chicken or beef stir-fry with noodles
- grilled chicken breast with vegetables or salad
- grilled Tandoori chicken with vegetables and chickpeas
- green bean and chicken curry (no cream)
- barbecued chicken and vegetable kebabs
- barbecued lamb fillets with salad and bread
- lamb fillet with couscous and green vegetables
- curried lamb, beef or chicken with rice and vegetables
- roast lamb, beef or turkey with assorted vegetables
- lean beef with steamed vegetables and chickpeas
- chilli con carne with rice
- veal and vegetable stir-fry with rice
- seafood pasta with flathead and smoked cod
- sardines on toast with salad

- baked ling with jacket potatoes
- barbecued tuna fillets
- baked Atlantic salmon with salad and lima beans
- baked snapper with vegetables and crusty bread
- baked beans on toast with salad
- lentil and pumpkin risotto
- homemade vegetarian pizza with no cheese
- fried rice with assorted vegetables (use minimum oil for frying)
- vegetable frittata

Often you may think that your eating is quite healthy, and you can't understand why you are not losing any weight. You may have certain styles of cooking that use 'hidden fats': cooking with lots of olive oil (even though it's good for your heart, it's still fattening), butter, cheese or other high-fat foods. There are some simple things to look out for when preparing food that could help you make a big different to your body fat, without sacrificing the taste or the amount of food you eat. These ideas are designed to keep your fat intake down.

- Eat 3–4 Weet-Bix and low-fat milk for breakfast (less than 1 gram of fat). Compare this with a fast food breakfast, which contains about 30 grams of fat.
- Don't use margarine, butter or cheese in your sandwiches.
- Excellent sandwich fillings are tuna in spring water, turkey and low-fat ham.
- Keep away from foods preserved in oil.
- Drink clear broths or vegetable soups.

- Make mashed potato with a little milk and a small amount of salt. Don't add cream, butter or oil.
- Bake potatoes and vegetables without saturating them in oil.
- Don't add butter to your potatoes.
- Use salad dressings that are nearly fat-free or make a vinaigrette.
- Eat avocados sparingly.
- Don't add cream to pasta sauces or soups. Imagine if you had to drink all that cream.
- Use lean meat, especially when you are making meat sauce for pasta. Remember that the meat will contain some fat so you do not need to add oil.
- Accompany pasta with a salad or some steamed vegetables. This will force you to eat less pasta.
- Barbecued fish or meat with salad is a great, easy-to-cook meal.
- If you have to use coconut flavors, use light coconut milk, not cream.
- Stay away from foods such as schnitzels that involve even the slightest amount of frying. This includes veal parmigiana, which contains about 40 grams of fat alone.
- Add some chilli to your dish. The capsaicin will increase your metabolism momentarily.
- Drink eight glasses of water a day.
- Buy a juicer and drink more fresh juices such as apple and carrot. The benefits and reported cancer-fighting

properties of vitamin A found in carrots look promising.

- Stay away from soft drinks; drink water instead.
- Never shop at the supermarket when you are hungry.
- Plan your meals for the week.
- Cook in bulk at the weekend and freeze some meals.
- Cook food in a slow cooker that you can set before going to work and has the food (such as roast) ready when you return.

SNACK ALTERNATIVES

- high-fibre/low-fat muffins, cookies or scones
- high-fibre/low-fat cakes such as carrot or banana
- low-fat/low-sugar breakfast cereals
- vegemite on toast (no butter)
- low-fat/low-sugar custard or yoghurt
- wholewheat biscuits with vegemite
- bruschetta (using wholemeal bread)
- small can of salmon or tuna
- 99 per cent fat-free crackers
- rice crackers
- muesli bars
- bagels
- glass of Sustagen
- baked beans (on toast)
- very small serve of pasta
- soups (canned)
- half a banana sandwich
- fat-free popcorn

- bananas or any other fruit
- flavoured rice pudding
- handful of raisins
- handful of sultanas
- a handful of Snakes, no more than once every two days
- a handful jelly babies, no more than once every two days
- Turkish delight, every second day
- Milky Way, every second day

EATING AT WORK

- Make your lunch before you go to work.
- Keep plenty of good low-fat snack foods at work.
- Use the microwave oven and cooking facilities at work.
- Don't make food that you won't eat.

Seven successful strategies to strip fat

1   Reduce fat to below 41 grams for women and 60 grams for men.

2   Eat four to five pieces of fruit every day (to increase fibre).

3   Eat fish once or twice a week (or consume fish oils every two to three days).

4   Eat legumes at least once a week.

5   Consume servings of brightly coloured vegetables each day.

6   Eat vegetable soup twice a week.

7   Reduce alcohol consumption and increase water consumption (6–8 glasses per day).

For women, optimise your calcium intake, with reduced-fat milk, reduced-fat yoghurt and fish with edible bones, and ensure that your iron and folate requirements are met by eating plenty of grains, cereals and meat (two to three times per week).

In summary

Never eat until you are full. This is a habit many of us have, but it is possible to break it. Keep your fat intake down and increase the amount of fibre you eat: four to five pieces of fruit each day will help you achieve this. Try to eat fruit, salad or vegetables before your main meals during the day. This will help keep your appetite under control. And remember always to have healthy food to hand to stave off bingeing on junk food.

CHAPTER 4

SEVEN DAYS TO STRIP FAT

Key messages for this chapter

YOU WILL DISCOVER:

- fat loss is enhanced when you decrease fat and increase fibre
- fat loss needs to be viewed in both long- and short-term goals
- exercise can boost fat loss
- how to map out your eating each day in advance

How to strip fat

To use the fat that is stored around your body you need to tap into your fat reserves. There is no point in using some fat, and then storing a lot. As we know, fat can be stored very easily; 97 per cent of the fat you eat is stored. The aim is to keep your fat intake very low. By doing this you will force your body to use more fat from around your body. This is the first step in using your body fat for fuel. Don't expect to lose 30 kilograms in thirty days. The body just doesn't operate that way unless you are in starvation mode, losing lean fat-burning muscle. With the 7×7 Fat-Reducing Plan, you will begin to reduce fat from your body after only seven days. And you can lose 8–10 kilograms of permanent body fat in twelve weeks.

By following the 7×7 Fat-Reducing Plan, you ensure that 55 per cent of your diet is from complex carbohydrates, and your body will begin to use its stores of body fat much more effectively. This works in two ways. Firstly, after you have eaten bread, rice, pasta or cereals you feel full, whereas when you eat fatty foods, you only feel more hungry. So you actually eat less food when the bulk of your diet is made up of carbohydrates. Secondly, in order to digest, transport and store complex carbohydrates the body uses three times more energy than it does for fat. The energy that the body uses to store complex carbohydrates comes from your fat stores! So the more complex carbohydrates you eat, the less fat you store and the more fat your body uses for fuel.

The third way to reduce your body fat is by stopping eating

before you are full. Don't roll off your chair after you have filled every ounce of space in your stomach. We all do that too often. Eat less, more often.

Ideal weight

A good way to work out your ideal weight is to measure your body mass index (BMI). This gives you the proportion of your height to weight. To work out your BMI, divide your weight by your height (in metres) squared.

$$\frac{82}{(1.75 \times 1.75)} = \frac{82}{3.06} = {>}26.8$$

The aim is to obtain a value of 25 or less.

BODY MASS INDEX (BMI) VALUES

<20	underweight
20–25	normal
>25	overweight
30–35	obese
>35	dangerously obese

Jan's last effort

Jan has been trying to lose weight for a long time, but like most people she travels along the rollercoaster ride of weight loss followed by weight gain. This is because most people lose water and muscle and very little fat. Fat loss requires a lot more thought and understanding. Jan is 1.62 m tall and weighs 67 kilograms (BMI 25.5) and although she doesn't look like she needs to lose weight she insists she does; not much, but she believes that losing 5–6 kilograms would make her happy. It would make her feel and look better. There is a catch, however: Jan wants to lose fat weight, and keep it off. The challenge is in front of her, just as it may be in front of you. If you are a few kilograms over your ideal weight, then you need to understand that fat loss becomes more challenging the closer you come to your ideal weight. For example, it will be easier for Jan to go from 67 kilograms to 64 than from 64 kilograms to 60. This is because the body tries to resist fat loss at various times. As the body loses weight, it expends less energy because it is carrying less weight around. This is referred to as the plateau phase. In this case you may need to eat different foods or cut down on your food intake. In the end, understanding and working with this in mind, it is a battle you can win. Let's see what she does.

For breakfast Jan has been having a bowl of 'normal' muesli, which unfortunately contains 8 grams of fat. Her first step is to change that to a high fibre muffin, with a scraping of margarine and a glass of orange juice. The fat in her new meal is only 3 grams. Jan hasn't eaten a big meal but she doesn't need to. The point of this eating program is not to eat until you are full. The fibre in the muffin helps her to feel a little fuller than if she had had a regular muffin, but she hasn't overeaten. The beauty of this eating plan is that another meal, although small, is just around the corner.

Mid-morning arrives and as expected Jan is hungry. Usually she would have a muesli bar and a yoghurt, assuming she was eating a healthy snack. Unfortunately the fat content of these two food options totals 11 grams of fat and has really been filling her up. Following the 7×7 Fat-Reducing Plan she can only eat two pieces of fruit (1 banana and an orange) during the morning. The fat cost is 0! Jan is advised to eat two different pieces of fruit every day. Variety is the key here, and eating a range of different fruits is not only enjoyable and tasty, but extremely healthy and energising. Eating two pieces of fruit fills her up just enough without making her feel as though she is bursting at the seams. Remember, we do not want to overeat on any meal. She also has two glasses of water, which should help to make her feel healthy. For lunch Jan would usually eat a cheese and salad sandwich (with both sides of her bread buttered), two chocolate biscuits and a soft drink. She has been eating 20 grams of fat in what looks like almost a perfectly healthy lunch. Chances are she has felt quite full. This is especially true for men, who must eat to capacity at all costs. Not only would Jan have felt full, her fat intake for the day would be slowly building up. As we have seen in the previous chapters fat contains plenty of energy per serving, two and a half times more energy per gram than bread or meat. By reducing her fat intake, Jan reduces the amount of energy she eats and consequently reduces the amount of energy she stores. In other words she reduces the amount of fat she stores and increases the amount of fat she strips from her body-fat stores. Following her new 7×7 Fat-Reducing Plan, she doesn't eat to capacity. She eats half a pita bread stuffed with tuna (which was canned in brine) and plenty of salad, especially green leafy vegetables, grated carrots, tomatoes and cucumber. She also drinks 500 mls of water. Her fat intake is 3 grams, and she is satisfied. The aim, remember, is to leave room at the end of your meal. This is subjective, so when you are starting this plan for the first time start small and build up. Your own metabolism may require you to eat three-quarters of a pita bread to make you feel only half full, and for a big man it may be one and a half salad and pita-bread servings.

Around mid-afternoon when Jan would normally start craving doughnuts, she opts for a small tub of low-fat, high-calcium yoghurt. The fat content is 19 grams for the doughnut and only 1 gram for the yoghurt. As Jan finishes work she is also encouraged to eat a piece of fruit, just to keep her going until dinner time. This is only a small meal, but it is essential to stop her snacking on potato cakes, chocolate and other junk food on the way home. (Once again, if you find that this is not satisfying enough, eat two pieces.) Usually for dinner Jan would have a piece of grilled fish with butter sauce, cauliflower with cheese on top, and other baked vegetables splashed with oil. Although healthy, the fat content is very large and can amount to 22 grams of fat. Her alternative is to have a small piece of fish with no butter but some freshly squeezed lemon juice, and some steamed vegetables, which include potato, pumpkin, broccoli and spinach. She may also have a piece of wholemeal bread. She doesn't eat until she is full.

When she first tries eating according to these rules, it takes a lot of adjusting, but she steadily adapts to eating smaller portions. Her fat intake is just 17 grams, which includes a teaspoon of healthy extra-virgin olive oil on her vegetables. The big change here is she has her steamed vegetables first, before her piece of fish. This is more likely to result in Jan eating all her vegetables, and less of her fish. This pattern is essential for all main meals. Eat the salad or vegetables first and then eat your bread, pasta or meat. Once again make sure these portions of food are smaller than usual, take a little break between food types, and chew your food several times.

Usually after dinner Jan would eat a chocolate bar (12 grams of fat!), but following her new 7×7 Fat-Reducing Plan she has a bowl of fresh assorted fruit salad, which has zero fat grams. Let's now see the difference in her eating for a typical day.

JAN'S DAILY INTAKE

MEAL	FAT IN JAN'S USUAL FOOD (grams)	FAT USING 7×7 FAT-REDUCING PLAN (grams)	FAT SAVED ON 7×7 FAT-REDUCING PLAN (grams)
Breakfast	8	3	5
Mid-morning snack	11	0	11
Lunch	20	3	17
Mid-afternoon snacks	19	1	18
Dinner	22	17	5
Dessert	12	0	12
TOTAL	92	24	68

As the table opposite shows there is a huge difference in the way Jan used to eat and the way she now eats following the 7×7 Fat-Reducing Plan. There is not only a huge difference in the amount of fat – a whopping 68 grams – but there is also a massive difference in the amount of energy she consumes. This 68 grams of fat is nearly 2600 kJ of energy each day that she had been overeating. Jan is also not an active person, so this 68 grams each day accumulated and was stored as body fat.

To get your body to use this extra energy is very demanding. When we eat plenty of fat in our diets, stripping fat is an immense task. As we know, for women anything over 41 grams of fat is stored as fat.

EASY FAT LOSS

	FAT CONSUMED (grams)	FAT USED BY HER BODY (grams)	FAT LEFT OVER (grams)	TIME NEEDED TO BURN OFF THIS FAT	WALKING DISTANCE TO BURN OFF THIS FAT
Jan's old eating habits	92	41	51	160 mins	17 km
Jan following the 7×7 plan	24	41	–17*	0	0

*This 17 grams of fat is actually lost from her body.

As the above table shows, Jan needed to walk about 160 minutes each day covering about 17 kilometres in this time, just to burn off the fat she was unknowingly eating. Conversely, following the 7×7 Fat-Reducing Plan she eats

24 grams of fat for the day. This means that *at least* 41 − 24 = 17 grams of body fat is used from her body each day. Remember also that to break down carbohydrates (such as the fruit and vegetables that she eats on the Plan), it takes three times more energy than to break down fat. This means that her body uses more energy from fat to do this, so she is using more than 17 grams of fat each day. Studies show that consuming a majority of foods that are of plant origin (as is contained in the 7×7 Fat-Reducing Plan) results in a resting energy expenditure increase of between 10 and 40 per cent. This means for Jan that she can use about 70 grams of fat each day from her body fat stores, resulting in about 500–600 grams of fat loss in just seven days. In ten to twelve weeks Jan achieves her goal of permanent loss of 6 kilograms of fat. She has reached her ideal weight of 60 kilograms and her BMI is a much improved 22.8.

Frank's Fat Plan

Frank has much more of a challenge than Jan, because men often overeat. We almost instinctively eat until we burst at the seams. How many times have you heard a man say, 'I'm stuffed', 'I'm full' or 'I couldn't fit another thing in'. How many times have you been to an 'all you can eat' restaurant and seen Dad, an uncle or even your husband go back for yet another serve. We usually call this value for money. In nutritional physiology we call this overeating and 'massive fat storage'. Overeating means an over-consumption of food, an over-consumption of energy, and weight gain.

For Frank it's not all bad, but he is approaching 88 kilograms and his stomach is beginning to take on a large, round appearance. Frank is 1.82 m tall and his BMI is 26.6. He aims to get down to 80 kilograms and, like Jan, he doesn't want to lose muscle and water, and rebound to an even greater weight after he has finished his diet. He wants to lose the necessary weight and keep it off. Whether you want to lose 8 kilograms like Frank or 18 kilograms, the principles in this book are the same.

Frank had always been very conscious about eating well. He had never thought that what he ate would lead to weight gain, until the weight appeared 'all of a sudden'. For example, for breakfast Frank would usually eat six pieces of toast (with margarine): two with peanut butter and four with strawberry jam. He had already eaten up to 16 grams of fat without knowing that this could be so bad. He then had a cup of coffee. Following the 7×7 Fat-Reducing Plan, he now eats three pieces of wholemeal toast, with a scraping of margarine and strawberry jam, a glass of freshly squeezed orange juice, and maybe a cup of coffee. He is not full but satisfied. To help with this change in eating habits, Frank chews his food more and eats it slowly. In days gone by, he'd barely have finished one piece of toast when another two would be in the toaster. The fat content of Frank's new eating plan is only 7 grams.

Like Jan, Frank has a choice of any two to three fruits at mid-morning. For many men this is a huge challenge. Of course, for Frank to get even half full he needs two bananas and an apple. But this is so much better than the occasional bucket of chips or bar of chocolate, piece of cake with coffee or waiting for the 'gorging session' at lunch time. The usual fat content of Frank's mid-morning binge is about 10 grams. This is compared to zero fat grams on his new Plan. Of course, there are men who will be half to three-quarters full with just one banana, and if this is the case for you, adjust the eating plan as necessary.

At lunch Frank would buy a pie; or some sausage rolls; or a chicken, lettuce, avocado and mayonnaise roll; or a roast beef, cheese, salad and mayonnaise focaccia. (He might have even taken some cream-based or olive-oil laden pasta to work that was left over from the night before.) Usually his fat intake came to 25 grams of fat because one roll for lunch was never enough: he had to have two. Not all men eat this way but many do, often on the days that they are inactive. It is very common to see fit people eat a lot of food and not get fat because they will burn all the energy from their food. Inactive people, however, should never overeat on any food. Following the 7×7 Fat-Reducing Plan Frank cannot overeat, but rather must leave room at the end of lunch because he knows he has an opportunity to eat another meal a little later. He eats a large tuna and salad roll, with no cheese or butter. He also drinks 500 mls of water. His fat intake is 5 grams. Once again he is satisfied but not full.

As the afternoon arrives he is hungry again, so he eats a low-fat muesli bar and a tub of low-fat yoghurt. This is much better than saving himself for an evening feast at dinner time, or collecting something edible and fast on the journey home.

Eating something fatty such as a potato cake, a packet of salt and vinegar chips or a small bucket of hot chips was a familiar story for Frank. His usual intake of fat at that time was about 10 grams. Now, just before he leaves work, he eats an apple.

For dinner Frank loved veal schnitzel, buttery mashed potato and maybe some vegetables. One serving of veal schnitzel contains 39 grams of fat. The mashed potato alone is fine but the added butter was giving Frank an extra 8 grams of fat. Frank's dinner was complete when he had his nightly bowl of ice cream – another 8 grams of fat.

Following the Plan Frank subtly changes his eating habits. He starts with a small bowl of steamed assorted vegetables. This is followed by a small bowl of pasta. These courses are spaced apart, so that Frank is not gulping down the last of

FRANK'S DAILY INTAKE

MEAL	FAT IN FRANK'S USUAL FOOD (grams)	FAT USING 7×7 FAT-REDUCING PLAN (grams)	FAT SAVED ON 7×7 FAT-REDUCING PLAN (grams)
Breakfast	16	7	9
Mid-morning snack	10	0	10
Lunch	25	5	20
Mid-afternoon snacks	10	1	9
Dinner	46	12	34
Dessert	8	2	6
TOTAL	115	27	88

one dish while preparing the next. Although rather satisfied, he is not bursting at the belt buckle. He finishes off with some low-fat ice cream with one-third less fat for dessert. His fat intake is 8 grams. He begins to feel lighter and much healthier. In the table on page 77, his fat intake is compared with his old way of eating and the new 7×7 Fat-Reducing Plan.

There is a huge difference between the way Frank used to eat and his new eating plan. As the table shows, there is a difference of 88 grams of fat between the way Frank used to eat and how he eats now; 115 grams of fat is a large but average amount of fat to eat each day. The male body will metabolise 60 grams of fat each day. This leaves Frank with a surplus of extra fat to the tune of 115 − 60 = 55 grams of fat. This is about 2000 kJ of energy that just sits in his fat stores causing him to gain weight. This 55 grams of extra fat that Frank has been carrying around each day takes an enormous amount of physical effort to strip or metabolise. People fail to understand that you cannot just sit around the house after a meal. Even a gentle walk around the block will not be sufficient to offset this massive fat load.

As the chart opposite clearly shows, Frank needed to walk for 140 minutes each day, covering about 13 kilometres, just to offset his fat load. Of course, this is just not practical to do each night. Following the 7×7 Fat-Reducing Plan Frank has reduced his fat intake to 27 grams of fat for the day. This means his body uses *at least 33 grams* of fat from his body fat stores each day.

EASY FAT LOSS

	FAT CONSUMED (grams)	FAT USED BY HIS BODY (grams)	FAT LEFT OVER (grams)	TIME NEEDED TO BURN OFF THIS FAT	WALKING DISTANCE TO BURN OFF THIS FAT
Frank's old eating habits	115	60	55	140 mins	13 km
Frank following the 7 × 7 plan	27	60	–33*	0	0

*This 33 grams of fat is actually lost from his body.

In fact the more time Frank spends on the 7×7 Fat-Reducing Plan, the more fat his body uses. Now that he's eating more plant foods and less fat, he loses as much as 70–90 grams of fat per day. In about ten weeks Frank has his weight down and his BMI is 24.1. Don't forget that our two friends Frank and Jan do not exercise. If they were to participate in some physical activity, their results would be even more rewarding. Nevertheless, they both reach their weight goals with only slight changes to their eating habits.

Exercise and fat

We have so far looked at what happens to weight loss, and in particular fat loss, when people follow the 7×7 Fat-Reducing Plan. As you are well aware by now, this plan encourages you not to overeat in a single meal or for that matter throughout the day. I understand that for many people trying to eat well and lose fat is challenging enough as it is, without adding more variables such as exercise to the equation. Having spoken to many people about this issue, it seems the greatest challenge is to first eat right. People often try to make too many radical changes in their life and sometimes these changes are too much too soon and are just not sustainable.

At some stage in the future you may hit a plateau with weight loss and in particular fat loss. In this case some form of physical activity will help you get over your plateau phase of weight loss. The problem for some people is that when they hit a plateau they eat less and less food. As we have discussed in the previous chapters, deprivation is simply not sustainable for a long time. How long can you not eat?

You may also just want to feel even healthier and fitter, in your quest for fat loss. This is where exercise can supercharge your metabolism, in combination with the 7×7 Fat-Reducing Plan. The most important point is to get the eating part right first, then look at some physical activity.

Many people think that just because they are exercising they can eat what they want. They believe their bodies will burn up most of the bad food or fat that they eat. This couldn't be further from the truth. The most fat you can lose over twenty-five to thirty weeks, without eating well, is about 1–2 kilograms of weight – even when exercising three to four times a week. This was found by a study that examined all exercise programs where the participants thought that they could eat as much as they liked and whatever they liked because they thought they were burning it all off. How wrong people can be.

Kim's quest

Kim has decided that she wants to lose fat from her body, but she wants to accelerate this process by doing some exercise. She wants to lose 5 kilograms as well as tone up. The challenge is that the less weight a person has to lose, the harder it is to get their fat levels down. Now the difference here is that Kim wants to lose fat, not weight. Weight loss essentially means that people lose water and muscle, and so when they go back to eating normally the fat stacks straight back on. Often you end up putting on more weight than before you started. Kim wants to lose fat, which means permanent fat loss.

As we have already seen with Jan, it takes ten to twelve weeks to permanently lose 6 kilograms of fat without exercising. After this time, Jan's total weight loss is 7–7.5 kilograms, of which 6 kilograms is fat (she actually loses more weight than 6 kilograms because as you lose primarily fat, you do lose a little muscle and water, but not a large amount). You would expect Kim to lose 5 kilograms much faster than Jan, as she is furthering her body's fat-stripping potential by doing some fat-burning exercise. Some people may want to get ready for a reason such as a wedding, summer or a holiday, and hence choose to reduce their body fat faster. This is where exercise is a bonus.

As I have already stated, the human body has to use two and a half times more energy digesting, absorbing, and storing plant food than it has to for fat (this process is called 'thermogenesis'). This is the first advantage that Kim has; on the

7×7 Fat-Reducing Plan her body will burn a lot of fat energy. She will save about 50 grams of fat a day that she would otherwise normally eat. (Remember that the average Australian, American or British woman eats about 70–80 grams of fat each day, and the average female body burns up only 41 grams!) Her next task is to strip fat even further from her fat stores. Let's look at Kim's seven days.

FAT LOSS IN SEVEN DAYS

DAY	FAT USED BY FOLLOWING 7×7 FAT-REDUCING PLAN (grams)	EXERCISE (walking)	FAT USED DURING THIS EXERCISE (grams)	TOTAL FAT USED FOR THE DAY (grams)
MON	70	60 minutes	15	85
TUES	70			70
WED	70	60 minutes	15	85
THURS	70	60 minutes	15	85
FRI	70			70
SAT	70			70
SUN	70	60 minutes	15	85
TOTAL	490	260 minutes	60	550

As the above table shows, Kim changes her body into a machine that burns fat much more efficiently than if she just ate well. The physiological adaptations to exercise, which includes fat-metabolising properties, are enormous.

By sticking to her 7×7 Fat-Reducing Plan, Kim allows her

body to burn about 70 grams of fat each day. This fat comes from her body fat stores. Unlike other programs, this 70 grams each day doesn't come primarily from muscle or water. Kim's eating is so important because many people believe that while exercising they can eat what they want and as much as they want. Wrong! As you have seen throughout this book, it would take the average Australian, American or British woman over 130 minutes each day to burn up the fat they eat. Doing aerobics for 60 minutes each day burns up only 15–20 grams of fat. This leaves another 70 (130 – 60 = 70) minutes of exercise to burn the rest of the fat.

On the weekends, although sometimes it is difficult to eat well, Kim learns to eat only until she is half full, never to

INCREASED FAT LOSS IN SEVEN DAYS

DAY	FAT USED BY FOLLOWING 7×7 FAT–REDUCING PLAN (grams)	EXERCISE (walking)	FAT USED DURING THIS EXERCISE (grams)	TOTAL FAT USED FOR THE DAY (grams)
MON	70	60 minutes	20	90
TUES	70	60 minutes	20	90
WED	70	60 minutes	20	90
THURS	70	60 minutes	20	90
FRI	70			70
SAT	70			70
SUN	70	60 minutes	20	90
TOTAL	490	300 minutes	100	590

capacity. As the table on page 82 also shows, she manages to walk for 60 minutes four times during her seven days. This uses a further 15 grams of fat each day for four days resulting in a total fat loss for the week of 550 grams. As she gets fitter and continues to walk in the coming weeks, her 15 grams of fat loss per 60 minutes increases to about 20 grams of fat. The fitter you become, the more fat your body will burn. So if we were to factor in this extra fat-burning potential, and the fact that in four weeks Kim can walk much further in her 60 minutes, our table would look even more inspiring.

Don't be daunted by the prospect of so much walking. Kim spends energy doing incidental activities (such as taking the stairs instead of the lift) at least two days during the week. Normally in the past she caught a train and a tram to work, but she decides to walk from the station, which means a 35-minute walk each way.

The table on page 83 shows Kim's week where she walks five times for the week and strips at least 590 grams of fat from her body fat stores. Although from a practical aspect some people would find it difficult to exercise five times a week, you must remember that Kim wants to accelerate her fat loss. This means that most weeks she walks three to four times, but there are weeks when she walks five times. Usually she walks five times per week three to four weeks in a row, and then cuts it back to three times. This keeps her motivated and she understands that she doesn't have to push herself hard all the time. Following this process she is not only able to cut 5 kilograms of fat from her body in about seven to eight weeks, but also loses a total of 6.5 kilograms of weight through small losses in muscle and water. Remember, conventional diets usually result in 5.5 kilograms lost in muscle and water and very little fat.

Greg's journey

Like Kim, Greg wants to lose about five kilograms not just by improving his eating habits but by getting fit as well. He wants the benefits of keeping excess body fat off his body as well as the numerous benefits of keeping his heart healthy. Greg is in a fortunate position because unlike most men, he isn't waiting to develop a weight problem before he decides to do something about it. He has watched his father put on weight and seen all the problems that go with being overweight.

Greg realises that, like many men, he is eating two and three serves each meal. He has no stop button to tell him when he doesn't need any more to eat. Once he ate twelve pancakes at a sitting and another time he ate one and a half family-size pizzas by himself. Although he is not an obviously overweight man, he knows that if he keeps on going the way he is he soon will be. For Greg the 7×7 Fat-Reducing Plan takes a little getting used to at first. He finds that he has been eating for the sake of it and most of the time he hasn't even been very hungry. Shifting his mindset to eat only until he is half full is harder psychologically than physically. Food to Greg means eating as much as he can, whenever he can. Food now has to mean sustenance without overindulgence.

Cutting out food like pizza with lots of cheese is an initial step, and getting Greg to eat more fruit and especially vegetables at night is the challenge. When his weight starts to go down, though, he finds this motivating.

He considers going to a gym to start his exercise program, but he has joined gyms before and after the first few weeks never returned. On previous occasions he went to boxercise classes, but once again, when the weather was a little cold, or he was kept back at work, he found that he couldn't be bothered. So on this program he returns to the most practical and sustainable exercise – walking. As a bonus he is able to take his wife with him four to five days of the week.

STRIPPING FAT IN SEVEN DAYS

DAY	FAT USED BY FOLLOWING 7×7 FAT–REDUCING PLAN (grams)	EXERCISE (walking)	FAT USED DURING THIS EXERCISE (grams)	TOTAL FAT USED FOR THE DAY (grams)
MON	80	60 minutes	20	100
TUES	80	60 minutes	20	100
WED	80	60 minutes	20	100
THURS	80	60 minutes	20	100
FRI	80			80
SAT	80			80
SUN	80	60 minutes	20	100
TOTAL	560	300 minutes	100	660

As the table shows, Greg has committed to a real lifestyle change in order to get rid of the developing fat on his belly. Although he is exercising five times a week during this quest for a leaner abdominal and lower-back region, he knows that realistically he can only manage three exercise sessions a week. He has made a pact with himself, however: once the fat is gone, he will maintain his healthy eating and take particular notice of the amount of fat he eats, and how much food he eats.

The table shows 660 grams of fat lost for one week, and in just over seven weeks he loses his 5 kilograms of fat. With this fat loss he also loses a little muscle, and a little water, resulting in a weight loss of 6–6.5 kilograms. Greg also adds some stretching to his program to stabilise and strengthen his lower-back region.

Dave the Dad

Like many people worldwide Dave the Dad doesn't really care about what he eats at this stage in his life. He weighs 112 kilograms. Ideally he would like to be 94 kilograms. Dave is thirty-four years old, married, has three children and has a moderately stressful job that allows him to leave home at 7.45 a.m. and get home by 5 p.m. He doesn't know that in 1995 4.5 million Australian adults were reported to do no physical activity. This is one-third of the adult population. The average amount of fat that men consume is about 100 grams. Of this 100 grams of fat, a vast proportion would be saturated animal fat. Apart from the obvious weight gain, there exists the accompanying risk of heart disease. Let's look at Dave's fat gain first during a typical week. A dietary analysis showed he has been eating 115 grams of fat on average every day.

Although the future forecast for this kind of eating is only a rough guide, Dave the Dad's weight gain would become a problem in only a short space of time. Continued eating like this would see him at the 120–130 kilogram mark within a year. At the time he realises that it's time to do something, there is already plenty of fat gain, and plenty of work to do. If Dave is committed and follows a reverse of his eating pattern for six to twelve months (low fat/high fibre instead of high fat) then his weight and particularly fat will reduce dramatically. Committing

INVISIBLE FAT STORAGE

DAY	FAT CONSUMED (grams)	FAT BALANCE	EXERCISE	FAT USED (grams)	TOTAL BODY FAT (grams)
MON	115	115–60=55			55 stored
TUE	115	115–60=55			55 stored
WED	115	115–60=55			55 stored
THU	115	115–60=55			55 stored
FRI	115	115–60=55			55 stored
SAT	115	115–60=55			55 stored
SUN	115	115–60=55			55 stored
TOTAL		385			385 stored

Total of 385 grams of fat stored for the week

for a long period of time with very good eating habits and exercise makes a huge difference. So in the next part of our case study we will show how Dave the Dad can go about reducing his weight slowly. If it takes 15 years to put weight on, it is not going to take just eight weeks to get it off. The mathematics just doesn't add up.

FUTURE FORECAST

TIME	FAT GAIN
1 week	0.385 kg
1 month	1.5 kg
3 months	4.5 kg
6 months	9 kg
18 months	18 kg

Dave the Dad starts by understanding that he consumes far too much energy (fat). If you remember that fat contains two and a half times as much energy as carbohydrates, then this is where he needs to make changes. Dave the Dad's body uses up about 60 grams of fat every day. This leaves Dave with $115 - 60 = 55$ grams of fat extra every day. If you were to use the Bilsborough Fat Cost chart to see how much time this would take to walk off, you would find it amounts to 150 minutes, covering about 14 kilometres. This is too much physical activity and simply not practical, so Dave needs to dramatically cut this food group down. If he can keep his fat grams down to 30 grams per day, during six of the seven days of the week, then this is a start.

DAVE'S INITIAL FAT LOSS

DAY	FAT USED BY FOLLOWING 7×7 FAT-REDUCING PLAN (grams)	EXERCISE COMPLETED	FAT USED DURING THIS EXERCISE (grams)	TOTAL FAT USED FOR THE DAY (grams)
MON	90			90
TUE	90			90
WED	90			90
THU	90			90
FRI	90			90
SAT	90			90
SUN	90			90
TOTAL	630			630

Total of 630 fat grams used for the week

Dave the Dad may not notice a minimum fat loss of 630 grams per week, but it's a great start. He cleans out his cupboard and has the full support of his family. Remember that Dave the Dad has a bit of fat on his body, so he burns up about 500–750 grams of fat every week. Dave the Dad continues this way for eight weeks and his weight goes down to 106 kilograms. Remember, all he does initially is cut down his fat intake and let his body do the work. And work his body does, losing 6 kilograms. He eats according to the 7×7 Fat-Reducing Plan (see Chapter 3) and never eats to full capacity. He always leaves some room and eats plenty of plant food. The loss of 6 kilograms of fat is very significant, and with this momentum and motivation Dave the Dad continues to face his challenge.

The next step for Dave is to start to exercise three times every week. If he can walk for 60 minutes or more, this will further boost his fat use, which he does. As the weight starts peeling off he also becomes more active with his children, playing soccer and basketball with them almost every night. The amount of energy he expends is huge. He also washes his car, takes stairs instead of lifts and takes up golf. This is called incidental activity because you are active without considering it to be exercise.

Dave eats small amounts of fat so his body can get the remaining energy he needs from his fat stores. He also further draws fat from his fat stores by exercising. Hence he has a double-pronged attack on his fat stores. Low-intensity exercise over a prolonged period (and this includes incidental activity) is ideal for fat burning.

The only thing he needs is patience. The longer he lets this process work, the more fat he will lose. In terms of fat gain and fat metabolism, this clearly shows what a person must do in order to burn fat.

In these twelve weeks Dave the Dad turns into Dave the Superdad, going from 106 kilograms to 95 kilograms. In the total twenty weeks he goes from 112 kilograms to 95 kilograms, a loss of 17 kilograms. Body fat measurements confirm that of the lost weight, 15 kilograms were actually fat. If Dave had dropped all his weight in six to eight weeks, he would have lost

DAVE'S ACCELERATED FAT LOSS

DAY	FAT USED BY FOLLOWING 7×7 FAT-REDUCING PLAN (grams)	EXERCISE COMPLETED (walking)	FAT USED DURING THIS EXERCISE (grams)	TOTAL FAT USED FOR THE DAY (grams)
MON	90	60 minutes	20	110
TUE	90			90
WED	90	60 minutes	20	110
THU	90			90
FRI	90	45 minutes	13	103
SAT	90			90
SUN	90	90 minutes	33	123
TOTAL	630	255 minutes	86	716

Total of 716 fat grams used for the week

primarily muscle and water, and he would have put that weight straight back on when he started eating normally again.

Dave has seen his BMI transform. At 1.88 metres tall and 112 kilograms, his BMI was 31.6 (obese) when he started the program. By week 8, at 106 kilograms, his BMI is 29.9 (overweight). At week 20, having lost nearly 20 kilograms, his BMI is a borderline 26.8.

Dave loses his weight in two stages: by dieting first for a couple of months and then introducing some kind of physical activity. It is common for weight to keep coming off simply by eating correctly; however, exercise introduced in the second twelve-week phase burns even more fat. Dave the Dad shows that weight loss and in particular fat loss can be achieved permanently when done properly.

Lisa and the 'corporate lunch' syndrome

Lisa is a busy person, very much entrenched in her work, but like many people she believes her life has balance. She's thirty-four, of moderate build and she thinks she's quite healthy. There are times when Lisa is flat out and work pressures push her out of her routine. When this occurs Lisa lets herself go: breakfast on the run, lunch at a restaurant and dinner in the form of take-away at a late hour. The fat content of foods eaten during these times is quite large if you don't take care.

These busy and stressful times are the times when you need to be at your best. You can get through these times if you find just five minutes a day to map out what you are going to eat and when you are going to eat it.

For example, if you are eating continually during the day because you have brought food from home with you, then when you eat out for lunch or dinner or both you are not going to eat massive amounts of food. Unfortunately if you let yourself go even briefly, that can be the catalyst that stops you from continuing any health program. Don't let the guilt that you often feel after breaking a diet or overindulging momentarily make you lose your motivation. A small hiccup will do little or no damage at all to your progress.

When we eat something that is fatty or sweet we may feel guilty. This is especially true when we are supposed to be following a diet plan. I spoke recently at a conference and when I suggested that *everyone* cheats while dieting, everyone acknowledged it and laughed. When we cheat or eat badly it feels that we have failed and that's the end of our diet! By understanding that one meal, one bad day or one bad week means nothing in the scheme of the long-term vision, we can feel better about what we eat, and ease these feelings of guilt. Let's have a closer look.

Lisa's bad week

Although Lisa hasn't made a conscious effort to eat well she also hasn't feasted on total fat. Her daily intake of 85 grams is still very high and will leave her with daily and weekly excess fat.

EASY FAT STORAGE

DAY	FAT CONSUMED (grams)	FAT BALANCE	EXERCISE	FAT USED (grams)	TOTAL BODY FAT (grams)
MON	85	85–41=44			44 gained
TUE	85	85–41=44			44 gained
WED	85	85–41=44			44 gained
THU	85	85–41=44			44 gained
FRI	85	85–41=44			44 gained
SAT	85	85–41=44			44 gained
SUN	100	100–41=59			59 gained
TOTAL		323			323 gained

Total of 323 grams of fat gained for the week

Lisa, like many corporate people, has gained 323 grams of fat for the week, as she has been unprepared and lazy in her approach to this particular week. The situation could have been very different if she had approached the week positively and made a real fist of it. Let's have a look. As the table below clearly demonstrates, if Lisa had kept up her routine during the more challenging times, she would have still lost a minimum of 546 grams of fat. Who would have given up during such tough times?

At B Personal we advise people that during the most challenging times 'you need to be at your best'. Fresh oxygen to the brain as well as plenty of good food will help you to think clearly and keep you functioning at your optimum level.

FAT STRIPPING IN SEVEN DAYS

DAY	FAT USED BY FOLLOWING 7×7 FAT-REDUCING PLAN (grams)	EXERCISE COMPLETED (walking)	FAT USED DURING THIS EXERCISE (grams)	TOTAL FAT USED FOR THE DAY (grams)
MON	70	60 minutes	15	85
TUE	70			70
WED	70	60 minutes	15	85
THU	70			70
FRI	70			70
SAT	70			70
SUN	70	90 minutes	26	96
TOTAL	490	210 minutes	56	546

Total of 546 grams of fat lost for the week

As the table shows, eating well even during busy times results in fat loss. Simple preparation and planning will help you to decrease your body fat and also, during busy times, decrease your stress and increase your productivity. When Lisa makes it a point to walk three times for the week, she ends up with a loss of 546 grams of fat for the week.

In summary

There are many reasons why we want to or need to lose fat and weight. Some people are told to by their doctor, and others develop motivation through other means. You have seen our four friends approach the 7×7 Fat-Reducing Plan through very different eyes. Whatever your goals are, you can see that there is always an adjusting period, probably more mental than physical. The end results are there for the taking. Fat loss through both fat restriction and not overeating is a powerful tool. Combining these two with physical activity is an even more potent and health-giving and fat-loss mixture.

As with all our friends in this chapter, fat loss allowed them not only to look great and feel fantastic but also to be healthy on the inside.

CHAPTER 5

THE 7×6
HEART PLAN

Key messages for this chapter

YOU WILL DISCOVER:

- what to eat for a healthy heart and weight loss
- suggestions for seven meals a day for six days
- our normal diet is conducive to an unhealthy heart
- eating carbohydrates will reduce your cholesterol levels
- reducing stress and anger will help your heart

Healthy hearts

One of the so-called luxuries of getting older is the joy of consuming the finer things in life. We believe we deserve foods of indulgence after a hard day's work or after a hectic week at the office. Gone are the days of sacrificing foods we crave, dieting and watching what we eat. In part this is very true, but what we reward ourselves with may be doing us more harm than good.

As children we ate as we pleased. There were no beer bellies, cellulite, weight gain or heart disease, and the boundaries on consumption seemed unlimited. As we moved from our teenage years into our mid-twenties things started to happen that we seemed to have no control over. The foods that we were so accustomed to eating although we knew they were bad, and that never seemed to affect us, slowly started to have visible effects. The fat started to accumulate, our friends became larger and their parents, uncles and aunts started to die from heart disease.

It has been known for many years that the earliest stages of heart disease commence when we are very young. In fact these early stages, called 'fatty streaks', have been found in the coronary arteries of children as young as five years old. As time progresses, it seems that our environment either makes them worse, resulting in heart disease, or masks their existence forever.

At my company, B Personal, we come across many clients who want to lose weight, and in particular fat. As part of our total package we firstly evaluate an individual's general wellbeing to prioritise health and weight loss. For example, in the last year alone 72 per cent of our clients have had to put fat loss second on the agenda, and put reducing the risk of developing heart disease as the number one priority. In most cases both can be achieved simultaneously. Many of our clients had one or more risk factors for heart disease. Risk factors are foods, lifestyles or habits that lead to damage to the heart and eventually an early death. Risk factors include:

- eating a lot of fat, especially saturated fat
- consuming too much cholesterol
- increasing your blood pressure
- becoming overweight
- developing diabetes
- smoking
- anger and stress.

Once these risk factors have been reduced, fat loss recommences or takes a greater priority. As one of our clients said, 'What is the point in being thin and dead?' Trying to achieve fat loss while harbouring risk factors for heart disease can be extremely dangerous. In many circumstances most people wouldn't even know they were at risk.

When we hear the word 'heart' we may be inclined to think 'men', but let me assure you, no-one is exempt from heart disease. Heart disease is the number one killer of people in the Western world. Over 1.1 billion people worldwide have the disease, with 12 million people dying annually.

You may never have given any thought to heart disease. There may be no history of it in your family and you may have very healthy blood pressure. However, the chances of you developing some kind of heart disease as you move from your twenties is quite high. One in six people have heart disease, and in years to come this could be one in five or one in four. You are never too young to begin looking after your heart!

Fat loss and reducing your health risk factors can go hand in hand. Remember always to work with your doctor. These practical guidelines will show you what you can do and what you can change in your lifestyle before you detect some form of heart disease or develop it further.

It has been strongly suggested that a reduction in weight of only 10 per cent in some cases can have very positive effects on heart disease. This can be achieved with diet alone. In order to achieve good results you must understand the energy cost of food (see Chapter 4). Fat, especially animal fat, takes a lot of time to metabolise. If you look at the Bilsborough Fat Cost chart you'll understand that eating something fatty like cheese means you may need to walk for a couple of hours to get rid of it, otherwise it gets stored, accumulates as cellulite and fat, and exacerbates your risk of heart disease. This means that cheese platters are definitely off the menu! A standard serving of cheese in a cheese platter can take above 160 minutes of walking to metabolise.

How much do I eat?

The eating plan is called the 7×6 Heart Plan and works on the idea of eating less, more often. It works on the same principles as the 7×7 Fat-Reducing Plan, but the focus here is on reducing the risk of heart disease as well as reducing body fat. It comprises seven meals per day for six days, or a 7×6 plan. This is a maximum food intake, and the mid-afternoon and late-afternoon snacks are optional. Now at first this may seem like a daunting task – seven meals in a day? However, there is some good evidence that 'nibbling' food has more positive effects than 'gorging' food. With long-term use there is a reduction in cholesterol and an increase in metabolism.

The eating plan that I have prepared for reducing heart disease is a general guideline. The meals themselves are designed to be practical but small. Fruit fills the spaces in between the traditional main meals. Breakfast, lunch and dinner are much smaller than usual, so you don't need to eat until you are full at these mealtimes. The portions that I've devised are not meant to be filling. You'll probably find that you'll feel just right after each meal or snack, and have enough energy to wait until the next meal to eat again. As you will notice with lunch, half a sandwich is very small, but if you have another meal at 2.30, the mid-afternoon snack, and again at 4.30, for the late-afternoon snack, you shouldn't feel hungry. This means that at dinner time you may not be hungry.

Of course, half a sandwich for a big man is hardly going to be satisfying. Use your discretion here: one to two sandwiches should be sufficient. The same goes for dinner, where your portions should be just enough not to completely fill you up. If you are becoming quite full after every meal, then either cut them right down or leave one of the snack meals out. Eating a large variety of foods is very important, so when you go supermarket shopping stock up on these foods for the week.

To create this eating plan, I've drawn on suggested consumption for people needing to reduce their body fat and improve their overall health. This regime is also drawn from recommended eating for people with high blood pressure, and for those who've suffered a stroke, heart attack or diabetes. Why not follow this diet to prevent all these health problems in the first place?

7×6 HEART PLAN

MONDAY	
mealtime	food
breakfast	2 high-fibre muffins with a scraping of margarine and vegemite
	1 glass of orange juice
mid-morning snack	1 banana
	1 orange or other fruit
lunch	½–1 salad sandwich or roll with spinach leaves, tomato and cucumber
mid-afternoon snack	1 small tub of low-fat yoghurt
late-afternoon snack	1 muesli bar
	1 apple
dinner	1 bowl of vegetable soup with 1–2 pieces of bread
dessert	fresh fruit platter

▶ TUESDAY	
mealtime	food
breakfast	medium bowl of oats with low-fat milk
	1 glass of orange juice
mid-morning snack	1 banana
	1 orange or other fruit
lunch	bowl of clear soup with 2–3 pieces of bread
mid-afternoon snack	1 muesli bar
late-afternoon snack	1 small tub of low-fat yoghurt
	1 mandarin
dinner	2 servings of legumes such as chickpeas and lentils, with rice
dessert	1 scoop of low-fat ice cream

▶ WEDNESDAY	
mealtime	food
breakfast	2 pieces of wholemeal toast with a scraping of margarine and jam
	1 glass of orange juice
mid-morning snack	1 banana
	1 orange or other fruit
lunch	low-fat Caesar salad with 2–3 pieces of bread
mid-afternoon snack	1 small tub of low-fat yoghurt
late-afternoon snack	1 muesli bar
	1 pear
dinner	seafood pasta (with fish rather than crustaceans) with steamed vegetables
dessert	1 small tub of low-fat yoghurt

▶ THURSDAY	
mealtime	food
breakfast	medium bowl of oats with low-fat milk
	1 glass of orange juice
mid-morning snack	1 banana
	1 orange or other fruit
lunch	½–1 salmon and salad sandwich or roll
	diet soft drink
mid-afternoon snack	1 muesli bar
late-afternoon snack	1 small tub of low-fat yoghurt
	1 bunch of grapes
dinner	small piece of lean beef with rice and
	2 different servings of legumes
dessert	fresh fruit platter

▶ FRIDAY	
mealtime	food
breakfast	2 pieces of wholemeal toast with a
	scraping of margarine and jam
	1 glass of orange juice
mid-morning snack	1 banana
	1 orange or other fruit
lunch	½–1 pita bread with roast beef and
	salad
	diet soft drink
mid-afternoon snack	1 small tub of low-fat yoghurt
late-afternoon snack	1 muesli bar
	1 apple

mealtime	food
dinner	grilled or baked fish with steamed vegetables
dessert	fresh fruit platter

▶ **SATURDAY**

mealtime	food
breakfast	banana smoothie
mid-morning snack	1 banana
	1 orange or other fruit
lunch	½–1 tuna and salad sandwich or roll
	diet soft drink
mid-afternoon snack	1 muesli bar
late-afternoon snack	1 small tub of low-fat yoghurt
	1 orange
dinner	grilled or baked fish with steamed vegetables
dessert	fresh fruit platter

One day off

On Sundays, you may prefer to relax your eating a little and you shouldn't feel guilty if you go out for lunch and eat too much. For the best results on this plan, try to eat small meals often during the day and choose from any of the meal suggestions from the rest of the week. If you do go out for a meal and want to ensure that you're eating as healthily as possible, see the eating out tables in Chapter 7.

Eating guidelines

The options for dinner are listed on pages 60–61. Remember that when preparing them it is essential to always prepare and eat the whole meal. In other words, don't leave out your salads, vegetables or legumes, as this is easy to do. I have worked with a chef to present some meal suggestions that you should find easy to make. This should give you ideas in combining foods, particularly the trickier legume dishes. If you find another way of preparing tasty legumes always make sure you keep the oil content low.

Some easy guidelines to follow are to keep the meat portions small and increase the salad and vegetable portions, and always eat the vegetable part of the meal first. Especially good meals for healthy hearts are:

- pumpkin soup with two pieces of bread
- steamed vegetables and mashed potato
- steamed rice and baked vegetables
- couscous and curried vegetables
- lightly curried vegetables and Hokkien noodles
- bean curd and vegetable curry.

The following sets of rules are completely incorporated into the 7×6 Heart Plan, but when in doubt you can always refer to these guidelines to see what you should and shouldn't do.

Rules for those with elevated cholesterol levels

- Increase fibre such as fruit, vegetables and legumes (chickpeas, lentils and red kidney beans).

- Increase complex carbohydrates such as rice, cereal, pasta and wholegrain breads.
- Increase physical activity. Walk three to four times per week.
- Use more olive oil, sunflower oil and soybean oil.
- Avoid saturated fats such as butter, cream, fatty meats, doughnuts, foods cooked in animal fats such as lard.
- Don't consume coconut cream or coconut milk derivatives. These contain palm oil, which can elevate cholesterol.

Rules for those with elevated blood pressure
- Decrease salt consumption.
- Decrease alcohol consumption to an absolute minimum or eliminate it from your diet altogether.
- Aim to lose weight, especially from your abdominal region.
- Never eat until you are full. Always leave some room.
- Use olive oil, sunflower oil and soybean oil but keep oil consumption down.
- Avoid saturated fats such as butter, cream, fatty meats, doughnuts, foods cooked in animal fats such as lard.
- Avoid coconut cream or coconut milk derivatives. These contain palm oil, which can elevate cholesterol.

Rules for those with high cholesterol/blood pressure and who are overweight
- Increase fibre from fruit, vegetables and especially legumes.
- Increase physical activity.
- Decrease fat intake, especially animal fats.
- Never eat until you are full.

The eating plan should be effective not only in improving your condition, whatever it may be, but also in increasing your weight loss. The group that has elevated cholesterol levels should lose weight on this plan, but the precedence is to reduce their cholesterol to healthy levels.

What to eat

The 7×6 Heart Plan recommends consuming foods from a variety of groups. This means that as well as reducing the risk of heart disease, you are also maintaining the optimal intake of vitamins and minerals such as vitamin C, calcium, iron, folate and zinc.

Legumes are very important in the reduction of cholesterol, and also help with an array of diseases including a reduction in the incidence of colon cancer. Chickpeas, lentils and beans are included in the legume group. They are high in carbohydrates and contain protein. They are also an excellent source of fibre and leave you feeling satisfied at the end of a meal.

To benefit our health on many levels, we have to eat four to five pieces of fruit each day. Studies show that fruit and vegetable consumption, especially by vegetarians, is associated with very low levels of heart disease. Fruit and vegetables also contain antioxidants such as vitamins C and E and beta-carotene, as well as carotenoids (see page 110). When you start on this eating plan, be sure to have fresh fruit in supply.

Antioxidants

A diet rich in antioxidants is suggested to aid in good health and defend the body against age-related diseases such as heart disease and cancer. Antioxidants neutralise the bad effects of oxidation. Oxidation is the process that occurs when a cell burns or uses up oxygen and produces by-products called free radicals. The free radicals can harm other body cells and tissue, contributing to arteriosclerosis (clogging of arteries), heart attacks, strokes and cancer.

Free radicals are assembled naturally in the body; environmental factors such as exposure to cigarette smoke or ultraviolet light can generate more. Antioxidants fight against free radicals and render them harmless. Antioxidant vitamins include beta-carotene, vitamin C and vitamin E. To ensure a bountiful supply of antioxidant vitamins in your diet, eat a variety of plant foods, including wholegrains, and seven to eight daily servings of fruits and vegetables.

Calcium

Calcium is important for the prevention of osteoporosis. Women especially need upwards of 800 mg of calcium every day. Men also start to lose calcium from their bones from about the age of 35. Cheese is a good source of calcium but as we have rediscovered, cheese contains just too much fat. We need the calcium without the fat. We can achieve this by studying food labels and eating the foods listed below. Consider that the average glass of low-fat milk has about 300 mg of calcium and a 200 gram tub of low-fat yoghurt has about 350 mg. Low-fat dairy foods such as milk and yoghurt allow for optimal calcium absorption. Good calcium sources include:

- skim milk
- yoghurt
- low-fat ice cream
- cottage cheese
- sardines
- salmon, canned
- dried figs.

Brightly coloured fruits and vegetables

This group of fruit and vegetables contains carotenoids. Studies have shown that a high consumption of brightly coloured fruits and vegetables is linked to a decreased risk of heart disease. These foods are abundant in beta-carotene, an antioxidant. Try eating a serving of green leafy vegetables, including lettuce and spinach every day.

Other foods in this group are apricots, mangoes, watermelon, cantaloupe, carrots, yellow and red capsicums and turnips.

Complex carbohydrates

This food group has many essential roles in the prevention of heart disease. Complex carbohydrates provide clean energy for the human body with no fat. Foods in this group should accompany your meat or fish dishes. They are stored in the body as glycogen and do not get converted to fat, so they are the perfect fuel for this diet. They provided the main source of energy for the Fat-Stripping Diet and the results for weight loss were exceptional. Include in your diet daily:

- porridge/oats
- mixed-grain bread
- wholemeal bread
- pasta
- rice
- corn pasta
- cereals.

BREAD, CEREALS AND PASTA

These contain no cholesterol, making them a great substitute for large amounts of fats and in particular animal fats. Foods in this group have been associated with cultures that have low levels of heart disease. These are considered complex carbohydrates. Other benefits: apart from helping your cholesterol profile, when eaten they require more energy to break down, transport and store than fats do. This means that they are ideal to eat as part of a weight loss program.

Fruit and fibre

Increasing the amount of fibre in your diet can have some fantastic cholesterol-lowering effects. In fact some reputable studies have shown a reduction of between 9 and 19 per cent of bad cholesterol. Try to increase your fibre to at least 30 grams per day (2 bananas, an apple, a pear, a bowl of cereal, and a bowl of wholemeal pasta). Fibre can be found in two forms, soluble and non-soluble. Eating soluble fibre leads to fibre binding to the cholesterol in your intestine. As fibre passes quickly through your body (as the body doesn't have the enzymes to completely break it down), it takes the cholesterol away with it. This leads to a decreased amount of cholesterol being absorbed and stored on your artery walls.

Eating plenty of fruit is extremely beneficial. The consumption of fruit during the day is mandatory for good health. It can also help in the cholesterol-lowering process.

Eat four to five pieces of fruit every day:

- apples
- oranges
- bananas
- mangoes
- pears
- grapes
- peaches
- plums
- nectarines

- prunes
- figs
- mandarins.

GOOD FIBRE SOURCES

A good breakfast cereal such as All Bran can be extremely beneficial. Foods such as legumes are also high in fibre and include:

- lentils
- red kidney beans
- lima beans
- chickpeas
- mung beans
- mixed beans.

Iron

The eating plan also provides plenty of iron for your needs. Women need about 12–16 milligrams per day and men roughly 8 milligrams. Do try to eat lean meat two to three times per week, whether it be in pasta or with vegetables; three-quarters of a cup of diced lean beef contains 4.1 mg of iron. If you are vegetarian or eat a lot of vegetables, include some vitamin C or ascorbic acid with your meal, as it helps the body absorb iron. Good iron sources include:

- lean red meat
- chicken
- fish

- spinach
- silver beet
- legumes
- cereals and grains.

Fish and fish oils

The good oils contained in fish are an integral part of the 7×6 Heart Plan. In Japan, there are traditionally very low levels of heart disease, and the Japanese diet is largely based on fish. For those who just cannot bear eating fish, I strongly suggest fish oil supplements, and in the eating plan where there is fish on the menu replace fish with lean meat, pasta or some other dish. Eat the following fish two to three times per week:

- cod
- herring
- gemfish
- salmon fillets
- mullet
- tuna fillets
- sardines
- mackerel.

It is important to eat the right type of fish. All fish contain the omega-3 fish oils but the oily fish contain considerably more. In some circumstances it may not be practical to purchase fresh fish all the time, in which case canned fish is fine. If you choose not to eat fish, you should have about ½–1 gram of fish oils per day. I also recommend that when you eat out, try to order the fish if it seems like the healthiest option.

FISH WITH NO CHIPS

A study of 852 men from the Netherlands followed their dietary habits for twenty years. It was concluded that those men who consumed fish on a very regular basis had a 50 per cent less chance of dying early from heart disease than those who consumed no fish.

The human body produces a substance called thromboxane (TXA_2), which tightens blood vessels and causes blood platelets to stick together. The sticking together of platelets is similar to when a scar forms on your skin, and such 'scarring' can promote heart disease. Fish oils produce a substance that does exactly the opposite of thromboxane – prostocyclin (PGI_2). This dilates blood vessels and stops platelets sticking together. In Western society we need to consume more fish on a regular basis to reduce tightening of vessels and thickening of platelets.

When Greenland Eskimos are cut they bleed for much longer than you or I would. This is because the fish oils promote bleeding, and stop scars from forming, or platelets sticking together. This is extremely beneficial in reducing heart disease because the first sign of heart disease is a 'scar' on the lining of the blood vessels. Preventing the 'scar' by eating fish will reduce the risk of heart disease.

Vitamin C

Like beta-carotene and vitamin E, vitamin C is an antioxidant. While beta-carotene and vitamin E destroy the free radicals in fat tissue, vitamin C zaps the free radicals in body fluid. Vitamin C also helps fight infection and helps keep capillaries (small blood vessels) and gums healthy. The average adult needs at least 60 mg of vitamin C per day. One medium orange or three-quarters of a cup of orange juice will supply that much. The body excretes any excess vitamin C through urine.

Off the menu

Pasta is one of my favorite foods. I like to cook pasta with olive oil but only a very small amount. All your essential fatty acids are contained in one tablespoon of sunflower oil and one teaspoon of olive oil. This isn't much at all, but this is as much good oil as we need each day. If you have elevated cholesterol, you can increase this amount to two tablespoons of sunflower oil and two teaspoons of olive oil per day.

So when making your pasta dishes, keep this in mind: some of you are going to have to cut down on the amount of oil you use! I have explained that you can have too much good oil in your diet. Any more than that and the excess good oil will get stored as fat. Over time this fat storage can amount to becoming overweight. You also need to cut out cream and cheese! Both contain saturated fat, which is usually stored around the body. If you are aiming to reduce your weight, then cheese and cream will make you store lots of unwanted fat.

Low-fat cheese is still high in fat. People say, 'But I need cheese for calcium.' Calcium can be found in so many other foods. The challenge is to make pasta without cheese and still make it taste good.

Sorry folks but this is the truth, as harsh as it may seem. At B Personal I find it difficult to convince people that olive oil, cream and cheese really are bad for them. Some clients tell me enchanting stories about how their grandparents lived to be 95 years old and all they ate was cheese, butter, olive oil and cream. Unfortunately we cannot eat the way our parents or grandparents did because we have many more luxuries than our grandparents. These luxuries interfere with the energy balance of our bodies so we eat the same amount of energy but don't expend nearly half as much.

Alcohol

Alcohol, particularly when consumed regularly, can increase blood pressure. In fact people who overindulge in drinking alcohol are those most likely to develop hypertension. To reduce your blood pressure, decrease your alcohol consumption to a minimal level or abstain completely. Too much alcohol can also lead to weight gain.

Cooking oils

Whenever you use cooking oils, use sunflower or olive oils. Whenever you are eating bread, use margarine, or an olive oil spread, but don't use copious amounts. The reason for this is that these oils have been shown to decrease your bad cholesterol. Remember that if your cholesterol levels are at a dangerous level, then reducing them is important. There is no point being thin with heart disease! Use only two tablespoons of sunflower oil or two teaspoons of olive oil per day (see page 116).

Salt

High sodium or salt intake is also associated with elevated blood pressure. To reduce your blood pressure, decrease your salt intake to extremely minimal amounts. Highly salty foods are usually chips, fast food and fatty foods. Cutting down on salt means cutting down on these foods.

Saturated fat

Reduce your consumption of saturated or animal fat. This includes butter, cream, full-cream milk, cheese, palm oil, coconut oil and fatty meats – they all contain saturated fat. These fats raise your bad cholesterol levels and decrease your good cholesterol levels. In particular pay attention to coconut products, which contain palm oil. Palm oil is used in the fast food industry and raises bad cholesterol levels. In other fast foods, including French fries, beef tallow is use. This is essentially animal scrap boiled down. Beef tallow is animal fat and, like all animal fats that we unknowingly consume, elevates bad cholesterol.

The heart

In the Western world there are risks with almost everything we do. There are risks when we cross the road, drive a car and swim at the beach. There are also numerous risks that we face with our lifestyle. What we eat, how often we eat and how often we exercise play an enormous part in the safety of our heart. In the last few years other variables have come into the equation. These include stress, anger and what we do to relax, if we get to relax at all. Our bodies absorb these variables and mix them with our predisposed genetics. The outcome more often than not is harm to our heart and an early, preventable death.

The heart is an amazing piece of human machinery. It beats at least 100 000 times per day, 37 million times a year, and over 3 trillion times in our lifetime. The heart needs to pump blood around the body so that all our cells get adequate nutrients, energy, oxygen and life. There are several things that you can do to interrupt this majestic internal pump. Although *any* of the factors mentioned above can increase the risk of a person developing some disease of the heart, genetics also play an important role. If your parents had heart disease, then there is a chance that you may develop heart disease. If your parents had high blood pressure, for example, then you may well develop high blood pressure. If your parents gain weight very quickly, then the same could be said about you. Have a look at what heart diseases your parents have or had, if they had any at all. Our genetics are a very strong indicator of our future health.

Other risk factors can develop because we choose to lead lifestyles conducive to bad health. For example, our jobs may be very demanding and stressful, and we may be working long hours, under extreme pressure. We may eat too much fast food, eat too much fat and stay put on the couch on a regular basis.

Usually heart disease means that the blood vessels that bring oxygen and nutrients to the heart become damaged. Like a flexible garden hose these blood vessels can stretch, bend, withstand huge amounts of pressure, expand when heated and contract when cooled. Consequently, like a hose that is not looked after, the blood vessels can burst under too much pressure, get clogged with junk obstructing blood flow, and wear away without warning.

How these vessels begin to deteriorate is still not clearly established; however, many factors are said to contribute. It seems that the earliest signs are plaques, or sticky substances like scabs, that develop and stick along the blood vessels (arteries). The earliest forms of these plaques are called 'fatty streaks', which line the wall of the artery and may result from the accumulation of too much saturated fat and cholesterol. Excess cholesterol in our diet is stored like pieces of garbage along the walls of arteries. This storage seems to be the site where fatty streaks start to form. As this mound of cholesterol grows, it narrows the blood vessels, decreasing blood flow to the heart. The link between elevated bad cholesterol and heart disease is so fundamental to health.

Think about this as fat loss with bonuses!

Cholesterol

Many people still do not understand that you don't have to be overweight in order for your cholesterol to be high.

In today's society, everything we do is assessed. Our performance at work is assessed, as is how fast we travel on the road, our finances when we apply for a loan or how much power we use in a month. On the other hand, we are often too busy to worry about our health, and alarm bells ring only when someone close to us passes away at a young age from a heart attack or stroke. How many of you know someone who has passed away from heart disease at a fairly young age? The first part of health assessment starts with your cholesterol. When was the last time you had your cholesterol checked; one month, six months, one year ago or never? Get your cholesterol checked regularly so you know your health on the inside.

Combining health and fat loss

In the early eighties, 1232 men were selected for a five-year study to investigate whether lowering their cholesterol and quitting smoking could reduce the risk of coronary heart disease. These men had total cholesterol levels of between 7.5 and 9.8 mmol/l. These levels are very high, as the recommended values on page 126 will show you. This study is commonly referred to as the Oslo Study. The participants in the study were asked to reduce their animal fat (saturated fat), and slightly increase their plant fats. These plant fats are called polyunsaturated fats and mono-unsaturated fats and include sunflower oils and olive oils.

For main meals subjects were asked to consume fish, low-fat meat, potatoes and vegetables. There was a reduction in the group's total cholesterol from 8.4 to 6.8 as well as a 47 per cent lower incidence of heart attacks. With time and a continued decrease in fatty foods, their levels were reduced below the ideal maximum cholesterol level of 5.5 as recommended by health professionals.

When trying to lower your cholesterol you need to increase your sources of plant food (carbohydrates, see pages 111–112) intake by about 10 per cent and use a little more olive oil and sunflower oil than usual. Why? Because the composition of olive oils and sunflower oils helps to reduce the levels of bad cholesterol, LDL. However, if these oils are the only fats eaten in your diet, then you should still be able to keep your fat intake to relatively small amounts every day. For example, you must keep your fat intake below 41 and 60 grams for women and men respectively. By doing so your body will devour its own fat for energy.

But your body needs good fats. It needs good fats called essential fatty acids from plant fat because the human body cannot make these fats. The human body needs one tablespoon of sunflower oil and one teaspoon of olive oil per day. This amount of good fat (about 17 grams) will be used for other important roles in the human body (see pages 23–25), but not storage of fat. If you have elevated cholesterol then you need to increase the amount of these oils you eat every day. If you can get 20–30 grams of this fat from these two oils and other plant oils, then you will not only keep fat off your body, but you will clean out your blood vessels. This means consuming only two tablespoons of sunflower oil, and two teaspoons of olive oil per day if your cholesterol is high.

Cholesterol is a waxy substance that is produced by the body. During a typical day the body can produce up to half a teaspoon of cholesterol. The body produces cholesterol because it serves important functions such as the production of sex hormones like testosterone, forms the structure of cells, and is used in making bile. Bile is responsible for fat absorption into the blood after a meal. When we eat fat, bile is released into the intestine and drags fat into our bloodstream. Remember, we need some fats in our diet because they are essential and contain fat-soluble vitamins. When cholesterol is produced (mainly in the liver), it is sent around the body where it can be put to good use. Any left-over droplets are then returned to the liver and recycled. As the body can produce cholesterol it is not needed in the diet. Plants, for example, do not need or produce cholesterol.

The transport of cholesterol particles around the body is done by cholesterol transporters, known as lipoproteins. Although there are many of these transporters, we will concentrate on low-density lipoprotein (LDL – bad cholesterol) and high-density lipoprotein (HDL – good cholesterol). The total cholesterol level is the addition of the good and bad cholesterol. Your doctor will give you these values when you have your cholesterol measured.

Low-density lipoprotein

In a healthy body the balance of good and bad cholesterol is maintained. Each cell of the body produces some cholesterol, as well as receiving some from the liver. Cholesterol produced in the body is sent out to the cells of the body from the liver, via LDL particles. Eating cholesterol-containing foods and any animal fat can cause a massive disruption to this balance. The body now has another huge load of cholesterol to deal with, from the diet. This disruption leads the body to find alternate ways of managing this excess cholesterol and the body searches for storage space amongst its cells.

As the body needs only small amounts of cholesterol, the cells stop producing cholesterol when there is excess in the diet. This is because at some point, the total cholesterol made by each cell and the delivery of additional cholesterol to the cell plus the cholesterol from the diet is far too much. It is simply not needed. Apart from these cells ceasing to produce cholesterol, they also close their gates, not accepting any more cholesterol from the liver.

The body now faces a classic case of over-supply, and little demand. What does the body do with all this excess of cholesterol? It can't burn it up so it must be stored. These LDL particles from the liver have nowhere to go. The food we eat keeps pumping these cholesterol levels up. So where does this excess cholesterol get stored? Well, it sits and accumulates like pieces of junk on the walls of the arteries that lead to your heart. The more of these foods you eat (and in Western civilisation we eat so much), the more you stockpile at the entrance to the organ that keeps you alive and gives you life. Think about your own diet and ask yourself, are you placing a strain on your body? Are you pumping fast food, copious amounts of cheese, fat, oil, chocolate, meat and animal fats into your body? If you are then you are putting your internal system under enormous pressure to perform.

With time, bad food choices and inactivity, your bad cholesterol will rise. This continual rise escalates your cholesterol levels into dangerous territory and hence you have the genesis of a risk factor for heart disease. Your heart is now at risk of stopping. According to the American Heart Association, 100 million people in the United States have cholesterol levels of 5–6.5, with roughly 40 million people with high cholesterol levels.

High-density lipoprotein

These cholesterol particles are responsible for clearing the bloodstream of stranded LDL particles and taking them back to the liver. The difficulty for HDL is that more often than not there is just too much work to be done. Often LDL particles far outnumber HDL particles. Generally speaking our HDL needs to be about 25–30 per cent of the total amount of cholesterol. With a careless food intake, lack of movement and cigarette smoking, the amount of these much-needed particles plummets to dangerously low levels. There are just too many bad cholesterol particles to be brought back to the liver. In more graphic terms, the amount of bad cholesterol piling up on your coronary artery walls is too much and with this stockpile always growing, HDLs fight a losing battle. The combination of high LDL and low HDL is a lethal combination.

Healthy cholesterol levels
You can obtain these values by asking your doctor for a cholesterol check. To understand your own cholesterol profile it may be important to know what are safe values are. These are shown below.

LDL	less than 3.4
HDL	more than 1.2
Total cholesterol	less than 5.0
HDL/LDL	more than 25%

In Australia 51.1 per cent of males and 51.2 per cent of females have their total cholesterol levels above 5.5. If your HDL/LDL (good cholesterol to bad cholesterol) ratio is more than 25 per cent, this is considered healthy.

Exercise
The only sure way to increase your good cholesterol is by exercising. HDL removes bad cholesterol from the artery walls and takes it back to the liver where it can be broken down. Exercising several times per week can therefore be extremely beneficial.

FOOD	TYPE	EFFECT ON LDL	EFFECT ON HDL
margarine/ sunflower oil/ green leafy vegetables	polyunsaturated fats	decrease	decrease (only slightly)
olive oil	mono-unsaturated fat	decrease	–
legumes/ fruits/ vegetables	fibre	decrease	–
butter/cream/ cheese	saturated fat	increase	–

Blood pressure

When was the last time you had your blood pressure measured? We focus on fat loss, but we may not understand that fat loss and blood pressure reduction go hand in hand, if it is done properly. This is another value-added bonus of losing fat properly. Understanding blood pressure is the key and is often not explained properly. In Australia 15 per cent or an estimated 3 million people have elevated blood pressure. What is blood pressure and how is it dangerous? High blood pressure is termed hypertension. This means that the pressure of your blood vessels is higher than normal. Elevated blood pressure is a risk factor for heart disease. In

Australia 30.6 per cent of men and 27.1 per cent of women have hypertension, and levels in Britain and America are similar.

Systolic blood pressure is the measure of pressure of the arteries when the heart pumps blood around the body. It can be compared to turning a garden tap on full very quickly and watching the burst of water race quickly through a garden hose. This pump of blood from the heart is very similar to the pump of water through a hose, and means that the arteries need to withstand enormous pressure. These vessels need to be consistently strong, but flexible, under the intense strain of blood flow. Just like a garden hose, a blood vessel, although generally strong, can undergo wear and tear under continual pressure. Medical science has deemed that a safe pressure of the arteries when the heart is pumping is less than 140 mmHg, or just 140 for convenience. Any pressure over this value means you have an increased chance of your blood vessel bursting, leading to some form of heart disease.

The second measurable pressure that we use to determine elevations in blood pressure is diastolic pressure. This measures the pressure of the heart as it is filling with blood. Let's say this value is 90 mmHg or 90. Comparing the two pressures is normally what doctors or trainers do when they give you your blood pressure readings such as 140/90. An elevation in the latter, diastolic blood pressure, is considered a stronger predictor for heart disease than in systolic. People are advised to keep this pressure below 85, as the table below shows.

DIASTOLIC	CATEGORY
< 85	Normal
85–89	High blood pressure
90–104	Mild hypertension
105–114	Moderate hypertension
> 115	Severe hypertension

SYSTOLIC	CATEGORY
< 140	Normal blood pressure
140–159	Borderline systolic hypertension
> 160	Systolic hypertension

In Westernised societies, blood pressure increases as we get older. However, in non-Westernised cultures this is not the case. Their blood pressure remains relatively constant as they age. Is there an environmental factor that leads to this blood pressure increase? We know for sure that genetics plays an important role in determining whether or not you develop high blood pressure. If one or both of your parents have high blood pressure, then the chance of you developing this risk factor is a good one. However, many other controllable factors influence your blood pressure. If you are aware of these factors, you can set about reducing your blood pressure.

Exercising three times a week, coupled with dietary restrictions, should reduce your blood pressure. This can also reduce body fat levels. Being overweight or obese is clearly associated with an increase in blood pressure. To reduce your blood pressure, decrease your fat weight. The reduction in bodyweight and body fat is the single strongest factor in decreasing blood pressure. Fat weight and blood pressure can be reduced together.

High intakes of fat and in particular saturated fat can lead to increased blood pressure. To reduce your blood pressure, decrease your fat and in particular your saturated fat. People with high blood pressure often have high cholesterol as well. This further increases your risk of heart disease. A decrease in abdominal fat of 5 kilograms can result in a decrease in blood pressure.

If your elevated blood pressure progresses to hypertension, you put your health at great risk. The amount of extra work that your heart has to perform puts the heart under great stress. By not controlling hypertension you risk injury to the brain, kidneys and eyes, as well as heart attack and stroke.

Stress

Often when we are stressed, we find that our blood pressure is increased or that we put on weight. One possible reason could be that during very stressful times, we let ourselves go. If one area of our life seems stressful, we might expect it all to come tumbling down on us. Reducing stress can help with blood pressure and weight loss. You need to be at your best when faced with stress. This means during these times you need to eat well, exercise and find some spare time to relax and do the things you enjoy.

Hormones such as adrenaline and cortisol are released into our bodies to help us cope when we experience stress. Prolonged chronic stress results in overexposure to these hormones. As time goes on, extended exposure to increased levels of stress hormones can be detrimental to our health. Chronic stress can adversely affect blood pressure, heart health, memory, and the immune system. Everyday stressors include:

- running late
- traffic jams
- job pressures
- family pressures
- forgetting important dates/times/items
- poor organisation
- lack of stress-relieving strategies
- poor diet.

Anger

Are you a little hot-headed at times? Do you find that more recently you are getting angry and losing your cool temperament? Well, there are links between high levels of anger and a higher risk of heart disease. An American study of 1305 older men revealed that those who were irritable, hot-headed and often felt like smashing things had three times the risk of heart disease than their mellower, less angry counterparts.

Expressing anger has also been linked to a higher incidence of stroke. One study showed men who constantly 'blew up' had double the chance of having a stroke than those who didn't.

Remember that almost everyone lives with stress. In fact it is how we manage stress that is important. You need to ask yourself what measures you have in place that reduce the amount of stress in your life. To combat chronic stress:

- get plenty of exercise (at least 30–60 minutes most days)
- get seven to eight hours of sleep per night
- write everything down in a diary, no matter how trivial it may seem, so you don't forget
- clean up and organise your work area
- prepare for the next day the night before
- eat well
- do some yoga or meditation
- do a pump or boxercise class to release some stress
- remember to laugh, share a joke and watch something funny regularly.

Another effective stress-buster is making sure you set aside some time each day to nurture yourself. Do things you like to do: read a book (even if it is just a couple of pages), laugh, listen to music, meditate, garden or paint a picture. Don't get used to sitting in front of the television and judging time by your television programs.

In summary

It is possible and extremely practical to reduce your cholesterol and reduce fat weight at the same time. The problem that I see everywhere is that we only focus on fat loss without all the other bonuses. Fat loss and reducing cholesterol can be achieved together and help you enjoy life longer.

CHAPTER 6

LOSE FAT AND LIVE LONGER!

Key messages for this chapter

YOU WILL DISCOVER:
- you should have your cholesterol levels checked regularly
- you should have your blood pressure checked regularly
- fat loss can go hand in hand with lowering cholesterol and blood pressure
- reducing the risk of heart disease should take precedence over weight loss

Corporate Karen's journey

As you will see with our friend Corporate Karen, in time you can lose a lot of fat while taking care of your health. When I met Karen she weighed 90 kilograms, and she was very depressed about her weight. She's a former corporate executive and now a mum of two. Like many people she had tried different methods to lose weight; sometimes she was successful but every time she stopped her diet the weight came tumbling back on. For example, she would be very strict for ten weeks, but one day after her diet she just had to cut loose. Her weight would fluctuate from 90 kilograms to 87 kilograms and then back to over 90 kilograms. She had her second child two years ago and was really concerned about her weight. Although she couldn't say for sure, she thinks she put on over 20 kilograms in two and a half years. This may seem like quite a bit of weight but this 20 kilograms is 22 grams of fat stored every day.

I dare say, though, that Karen's fat gain would have commenced well before her pregnancy. Being a corporate woman, all her office lunches and dinners at various functions, combined with eating out because she'd finish work late, would definitely have caused fat storage. Like many people she'd also not eat during the day if she knew she was going out for dinner at her favourite restaurant. Once there she would gorge until she was very full. Entrées, main course, creamy desserts, wine and, to top it all off, a cheese platter. 'What's wrong with a little cheese?' she'd ask. When I asked her to show me how much her idea of 'a little cheese' was, it amounted to 42 grams of fat, which would take 140 minutes of walking, covering 14.5 kilometres. It was quite common for Karen to eat cheese like this three to four times per week, like many people.

I asked her why she stopped following her previous diets after only ten weeks and why she hadn't continued with them for six months. She told me that they were so difficult to maintain that after ten weeks she was exhausted both physically and mentally. On several different occasions she recalled being at a barbecue on a Sunday and while everyone else ate and drank as they pleased, she would just eat salad and hate herself for it. Another time she went out for dinner and threw her diet away after not having the faintest idea how to order foods in the specific ratio that her diet at the time told her to. She was sick and tired of always feeling hungry, some-times eating only fruit, and having no energy. She would feel faint on the odd occasion because she just didn't eat enough food. Dieting was a torturous experience. It took so much willpower but in the long term yielded no long-term results. This is when she contacted me, in a last-ditch effort to do something about her weight.

At 90 kilograms and 1.62 m in height Karen is categorised as obese. Her BMI is 34.3. We could just start her on a training program to reduce her body fat, but there are other factors that may be important to her health. If Karen starts a fat-loss program without checking up on what I call her 'inner health', then she could exacerbate these problems further, if they exist.

Some of these 'inner health' problems could be elevated cholesterol levels or high blood pressure.

The first step is to work with her doctor to develop a medical profile on her health characteristics as well as measure her percentage of body fat and the amount of muscle on her body. We can then test these values again in eight to twelve weeks' time and monitor her progress. She is primarily focusing on her weight loss and in particular fat loss, but it is essential to monitor all aspects of her health. This is something that I urge anyone to do when losing weight.

Karen's profile shows that even though she primarily wants to address the issue of being overweight, she also has the following health concerns:

- high cholesterol levels
- elevated blood pressure.

KAREN'S PRE-DIET RESULTS

Weight	90 kg
Percentage body fat	38%
Fat weight	34.2 kg
Muscle (fat-free) weight	55.8 kg
BMI	34.3
Blood pressure	145/87
Cholesterol	6

Karen also has her body fat percentage measured. This box shows that her percentage body fat is also very high and this needs to be monitored, as small changes in this value over a period of time are very significant and motivating. By constantly measuring a variety of aspects, Karen gets to see for herself whether her program is working or not. The fact that she has been inactive for most of her life hasn't helped her situation, but she is determined to give this a real go. Let's see how she fares.

In order to reduce her body fat, Karen has to cut down on the amount of fat that she consumes, which we calculate at about 95 grams per day. This means that every day Karen would consume 54 grams more fat than her body could use (95 − 41 = 54 grams). It would take her 175 minutes of walking (19 kilometres) just to burn off this fat. Karen's source of fat is cheese, cakes, biscuits, chocolate and ice cream. What she doesn't realise is that there are also hidden fats in much of the food she eats, particularly in restaurants. Like many people, Karen doesn't really know what is in the foods she eats away from home.

So she cuts out cheese, creamy desserts, potato chips and her daily bar or two of chocolate. She also eliminates saturated fats, which can elevate her cholesterol. She obtains her calcium from low-fat, high-calcium milk and yoghurt, and cuts down her salt. She also replaces her fat with fibrous foods: more fruit, vegetables, grainy bread, rice and pasta.

When Karen began to change her eating program, she put a lot of blame on herself and said that she ate too much food. Don't be so harsh on yourself! If you have tried to lose weight by following fad diets, how are you to know what is the most effective and permanent way to lose fat? People can reduce the amount of food they eat but still consume the wrong type of food, therefore still retaining or storing fat. It is therefore very important to have a look at how much fat you are eating every day and how much food.

An extra 22 grams of fat every day has lead to Karen gaining over 20 kilograms in two and a half years. This is the equivalent of eating one of the following every day:

- 1 tablespoon of margarine and ½ tablespoon of cooking oil
- a slice of chocolate cake
- 2 very small pieces of cheese
- 2 grilled sausages.

Although these amounts seem very harmless on the surface, they in fact mean just a little too much fat eaten for the day. Making these small changes can have very large implications.

On her new eating program Karen's total fat for the day doesn't usually exceed 1 tablespoon of sunflower oil and 1 teaspoon of olive oil, with 1–2 grams of omega-3 fish oils every second day. All this fat will not get stored as fat but rather go towards other roles in the body such as cell structure and hormone production.

While her cholesterol levels are still high, Karen has increased her intake of sunflower oil and olive oil. Remember, these oils help to reduce cholesterol levels. These are increased to 2 tablespoons of sunflower oil and 2 teaspoons of olive oil and in Karen's particular situation this is essential, otherwise she will need to go on medication. Her salt intake is decreased and she has never consumed alcohol on a regular basis so weight reduction is the only other variable needed to reduce her blood pressure.

Short-term goals

Karen's aim is to get through the first eight weeks changing her eating so that she consumes only three fat sources – sunflower oil, olive oil and omega-3 fish oil – for the day. Following the 7×6 Heart Plan and then the 7×7 Fat-Reducing Plan (see Chapter 3), this means that she has to totally clean out her existing cupboards of all products such as:

- full-cream milk
- butter
- cheese
- cream and ice cream
- tuna in oil
- sardines in oil
- peanut butter (that she used to finish in less than a week by herself)
- chocolate biscuits
- corn chips
- chocolate bars (cut down to one bar every two days, but not solid chocolate)
- cheesecakes

- packet cake mixes
- fatty mince
- packets of salted peanuts and cashew nuts.

Interestingly enough, many of these food items are very common in normal households, not just Karen's. Whenever I help people with their diets I always ask to look in the pantry, fridge and freezer. I can usually get a fairly good understanding of what a person's eating habits are just from this inspection. When a household is stocked full of high-fat foods the adults usually say, 'Oh, they're for the kids', or 'I don't eat a lot of it, I just eat bits and pieces.' In fact these bits and pieces are quite accumulative, and having foods there for the kids is your excuse to eat what you want. If this sounds like your pantry, then clean it out, if not for yourself then for the long-term health of your children. It's amazing how people will change the entire food pyramid that exists in a household once someone in the family has suffered a heart attack!

After the big clean-out Karen makes sure that the fat grams in all the foods in her pantry and fridge are very low. She clearly understands that you cannot overeat on low-fat products. She always knew about the nutritional labels on packets of food, but now she understands the importance of these labels. Her other aim is to prepare more meals from home and eat out less. If you have a healthy snack before you dine out, you won't eat as much.

RESULTS AFTER EIGHT WEEKS

Weight	83.6 kg
Weight loss	6.4 kg
Percentage body fat	35.5%
Change in percentage body fat	−2.5%
Fat weight	29.7 kg
Fat weight lost	4.5 kg
Fat-free weight	53.9 kg
Fat-free weight lost	1.9 kg
BMI	31.8
Blood pressure	136/80
Cholesterol	5.2

As the results show, Karen has lost 6.4 kilograms, most of which is fat weight. Needless to say, Karen is very pleased with her results but there is still some work to do if she is going to obtain further fat loss. Previously, if Karen were following a diet and lost some weight, she would go out and celebrate with some 'naughty' foods, and in time her weight would return. In this case she knows she can keep going. She celebrates by having her hair done and a massage, buying some new CDs and going out with friends to see a movie.

It's interesting to see that Karen has lost all this weight but hasn't yet started any exercise. In her quest to keep reducing her body fat she may need to eventually incorporate some exercise. When asked about the difficulty in maintaining this diet plan, she replies, 'Its easy.'

This setting of a short-term goal is important, as it gives you time to sit back and assess your progress. If things haven't worked, then why not? When things don't go to plan it's usually because people tend to cut corners, have the odd chocolate bar here and there or give up and start again several times during the diet. The problem here may not in fact be the person on the diet, but rather the diet itself. Some diets that expect people to survive on low energy for a long period of time are surely asking for non-compliance.

THE NEXT TWELVE WEEKS (TWENTY WEEKS IN TOTAL)

Weight	72.9 kg
Weight lost	17.1 kg
Percentage body fat	19.3%
Change in percentage body fat	−19%
Fat weight	20.15 kg
Fat weight lost	14.05 kg
Fat-free weight	52.75 kg
Fat-free weight lost	3.05 kg
BMI	27.8
Blood pressure	120/77
Cholesterol	4.7

During the next twelve weeks of her diet she includes a combination of 60 minutes of walking and 20 minutes of resistance training, three times per week. One of the main themes of metabolism that I have been trying to get people to understand is that if your eating plan is high in fat then exercising three times per week will benefit your heart, but it won't metabolise or burn up this fat. Weight loss in this case will be hindered. If your eating plan is low in fat then exercising three times per week will do plenty to further chew up your body fat. And fat certainly gets chewed up from Karen's fat stores, as her new results indicate. As the chart shows, she has lost over 14 kilograms of body fat in total, which is huge. The amount of fat she has on her body is only 20 kilograms as compared to 34.2 kilograms when she started. The double-edged sword of her new lifestyle plan also cuts her cholesterol levels, which have came down from the dangerous level of 6.0 to a very good level of 4.7. Her blood pressure is also much improved.

Putting the results of her whole program together indicates that she has comprehensively achieved a number of results beneficial to her health. She has not only cleared out lots of fat from her body, such as around her waist, the back of her legs and her bottom, but she has also cleared plenty of the fat that was being stored on the walls of her blood vessels, namely cholesterol. In very simple terms she has lost fat from her body, and cleared her blood vessels of the bad blood fat that we know as LDL.

The fat loss plan

Firstly, Karen follows the 7×6 Heart Plan. For the first few weeks, this is what her plan looks like.

STRIPPING FAT IN SEVEN DAYS

DAY	FAT USED FROM HER BODY BY FOLLOWING 7×6 HEART PLAN (grams)	EXERCISE COMPLETED	FAT USED DURING THIS EXERCISE (grams)	TOTAL FAT USED FOR THE DAY (grams)
MON	80			80
TUE	80			80
WED	80			80
THU	80			80
FRI	80			80
SAT	80			80
SUN	80			80
TOTAL	560			560

Total of 560 grams of fat lost for the week

If you have more fat on your body like Karen, then you are likely to lose close to 400–600 grams of fat for the week. Also there are some fantastic adaptations that the body undergoes to use more fat. In fact Karen loses 560 grams of fat per week, which is close to 80 grams per day.

Karen doesn't exercise in the initial eight-week period. To change her eating habits and make her exercise would have been too much too soon. This is the same for a lot of people who find it difficult to adjust to complete changes in their lifestyle. Too big a change is sometimes just too hard to maintain. For some it is easy for a while but the spark dies off. In other cases the motivation is here for a while but the pressure to maintain eating well and exercising like crazy for long periods of time becomes too exhausting and causes, oddly enough, an unbalanced lifestyle. The important thing is that Karen has a long-term goal so we can take our time and introduce variables slowly. What is the point in rushing to get weight down if it is only going to be for the short term, and then put it back on again?

As the chart shows, she strips an average of 80 grams of fat every day. On the weekend she could cut loose to some extent, but remember Karen has high blood pressure and high cholesterol levels, so she has to be careful. Even though she is very careful with her eating, she does indulge occasionally, which is fine. The 7×6 Heart Plan allows you to eat foods of your indulgences occasionally without feeling guilty. This is why diets like this are very sustainable in the long term. Karen uses the suggestions for eating out (see Chapter 7) to help her keep control even when she isn't specifically following the eating plan.

Karen then introduces some exercise into her regime. On the days she walks and weight-trains she is able to use about 600 grams of fat at the start. (In this twelve-week phase, if you cannot get to a gym or use weights, then extend this walking time, do some stair climbing and add some sit-ups.) On the days where Karen just eats according to the eating plan, without exercising, she loses roughly 80 grams of fat. On average for the days she is active, her fat use is bolstered to 90 grams of fat per day. This may seem small but it is a hugely significant increase.

The fitter you become the better the body becomes at using fat, so fat loss in a week can be around 600–800 grams depending on how your body responds to being physically active. Remember that during this twelve-week phase, Karen loses 10.7 kilograms of which 9.5 kilograms were fat. In fact Karen loses about 800 grams of fat per week, due to the increase of her exercise.

The wash-up

Karen is a very good example of someone who stuck it out. She has not only achieved short-term success through weight loss and in particular fat loss but also long-term fat and weight loss. Once this time is up it is important to maintain your weight and, equally importantly, your health.

Karen is a good role model for both men and women to follow. Too many people convince themselves that fat loss can only be achieved quickly or not at all. Other people think 'short term' and don't plan both short-term and long-term goals. Short-term goals are like a checklist to make sure that you are on track for your main long-term vision. Karen's eight-week short term shows that with solid changes and very little deprivation, good fat loss can be achieved. She is on track to achieve her long-term goals and this reinforces all the

KAREN'S ACCELERATED FAT STRIPPING

DAY	FAT USED BY FOLLOWING 7×7 FAT–REDUCING PLAN (grams)	EXERCISE COMPLETED	FAT USED DURING THIS EXERCISE (grams)	TOTAL FAT USED FOR THE DAY (grams)
MON	80	60 minutes walking & light weights	20	100
TUE	80			80
WED	80	60 minutes walking	15	85
THU	80			80
FRI	80			80
SAT	80	30 minutes light weights	5	85
SUN	80	90 minutes walking	26	106
TOTAL	560	240 minutes	66	616

Total of 616 grams of fat lost for the week

positive changes in her life. Like anyone who is committed and truly understands how the body uses fat you too can take 14 kilograms of fat off your body and keep it off. Of course, Karen could speed this process up if she had more time, but these days time eludes most of us, so we are forced to take practical measures, which means looking long-term. At B Personal we have achieved great results in both men and women following an identical program to Karen's.

Achieving your goals

You should find that by following either the 7×6 Heart Plan or the 7×7 Fat-Reducing Plan, after eight to twelve weeks you will have lost a substantial amount of weight without needing to exercise. After eight to twelve weeks, you might need to begin some form of exercise to keep up the momentum of weight loss.

If you're looking for the ideal exercise, brisk walking is it. This will cause your body to search for even more fat to use for fuel as well as make you respond to the numerous fat-burning adaptations of the exercise and your body will be forced to chew into your fat stores to get energy. Make changes in your life gradually; diet first, then exercise, then mix them together to get a lifestyle change.

James is under pressure

James is thirty-nine years of age. He's married and has three children. He is a stockbroker and works long hours and feels he is under a lot of pressure with his job. When James comes to us at B Personal he weighs 109 kilograms.

JAMES'S CHOLESTEROL PROFILE

LDL	5.2
HDL	1.5
Total	6.7
HDL/LDL	16%

This is a not a particularly good cholesterol profile (or blood lipid profile as it is sometimes to referred to). As the table clearly shows, James has very high total cholesterol, which also means that his bad cholesterol is very high. These are 6.7 (total) and 5.2 (LDL) respectively. Remember this is the cholesterol that gets deposited on the walls of the arteries. James's good cholesterol is dangerously low. Only 16 per cent of James's cholesterol is good, whereas this value should be around 25 per cent or greater. This means that more cholesterol is being deposited on the artery walls than is being brought back to the liver.

His doctor has told him that if his cholesterol levels continued to deteriorate, then he will have to go on medication. He has to elevate his good cholesterol and decrease his bad cholesterol. By increasing his good cholesterol levels he is recruiting more 'workers' in the blood to take bad cholesterol from the walls of the arteries and return them to the liver where they can be broken down. When we studied James's family, we found that none of his parents or relatives had high cholesterol levels. Admittedly James tells us he doesn't eat very well and is willing to do anything to get his levels back to a safe range. He has been warned by his doctor to make this his highest priority. James also wants to lose weight, so we have two tasks that we could achieve together. If he doesn't, he would be staring at an early death.

Some of James's changes

Just as Karen did, James has to make some significant modifications to his lifestyle. He cuts out all saturated fats and cholesterol from his diet. This includes:

- large amounts of meat and meat products
- butter
- full-cream milk
- cream
- cheese
- full-cream ice cream
- yoghurt
- eggs
- creamy soups
- creamy pastas
- coconut milk
- fried foods
- fast foods
- fatty meats
- lobsters, prawns, shrimp, oysters
- brains
- offal.

James also makes it a point to make most of his meals plant-food based and follows the 7×6 Heart Plan (see Chapter 5). He eats plenty of complex carbohydrates such as pasta, rice, polenta, and breakfast cereals. He never gorges on these foods, and after every meal he makes sure he isn't completely full.

I have assured him that in this process of reducing his cholesterol, he will also lose weight.

The no-nos

If your cholesterol levels are elevated, you will also need to abstain from this select group of foods during the next six- to eight-week period. All these foods have the potential to increase the levels of your bad cholesterol. Notice that seafood is in this list. This is what I call the seafood paradox: seafood of crustacean nature contains no fat but plenty of cholesterol. Notice also that we don't see carbohydrates on the list of foods that raise your blood fat (cholesterol). Yet, still some diet books claim that carbohydrates are bad for you, even though they are crucial in reducing your bad cholesterol (see pages 111–112). The majority of foods mentioned in the list on page 151 are very high in fat. By cutting or drastically reducing them you will reduce cholesterol and weight, in particular fat weight, together.

Stage two: testing James

Sometimes when your doctor gives you an ultimatum you just have to make changes in your life, whether you like them or not. I work with many people after they have had a heart attack. Their biggest regret is that they never followed my programs earlier. After following a rigorous cholesterol-lowering program for twelve weeks it was essential for James to be re-tested. Nine times out of ten, people's levels can parallel

BLOOD LIPID PROFILE

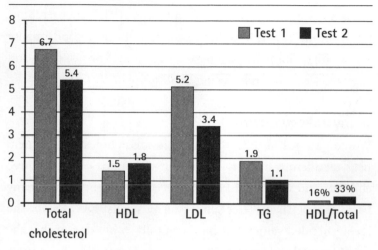

James's second set. As you can see, there has been a noticeable drop in James's total cholesterol: from 6.7 to 5.4, (–20%), the drop in LDL cholesterol from 5.2 to 3.4, (–35%), and the increase in HDL levels from 1.5 to 1.8, (+70%). James has successfully reduced his cholesterol to a much lower risk factor range. He is now able to focus more on reducing body fat, keeping in mind that if he were to eat badly in the future, his cholesterol levels could rise again. The great thing about what James has achieved is that he has also reduced his bodyweight down to 97 kilograms while focusing primarily on his cholesterol. His Body Mass Index is now 29.28. He's still in the overweight category but this is a much improved result.

One of the ways in which James has increased his good cholesterol is to walk three or four times a week for about

60–70 minutes. Walking not only increases good cholesterol levels and helps reduce bad cholesterol but also burns a lot of fat. In terms of eating well, the consumption of good-quality bread, high-fibre muesli, pasta, rice, and fibrous fruit and vegetables can aid in lowering cholesterol.

Jenny takes control

Women are just as likely to have elevated cholesterol as men. Let's take Jenny, a thirty-three-year-old mum who has three children and weighs 84 kilograms (BMI = 30.1). When Jenny first comes to us her cholesterol levels are above the recommended values. She has been told by her doctor that she should give this some attention. Just as James did, she reduces the amount of animal products in her diet to a minimum. She replaces these fats with olive oil and sunflower oil or canola oil

BLOOD LIPID PROFILE

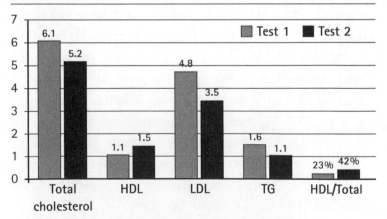

and increases her consumption of complex plant foods such as pasta, rice, cereals, wholemeal breads and vegetables. In just eleven weeks both her weight and her cholesterol have been reduced. Jenny also finds time to walk three times per week, by taking her children to school and picking them up on foot rather than using the car. This simple exercise reduces her weight to 75 kilograms in only eleven weeks (BMI = 26.9).

Blood pressure problems

Carmel met B Personal during a corporate seminar and discovered she had high blood pressure. This was something that her doctor had measured about eight years ago. At that stage she was fine so she thought she didn't have to get this measured again. This time, with the encouragement of her doctor, she opts to work with us instead of taking medication

CARMEL'S BLOOD PRESSURE

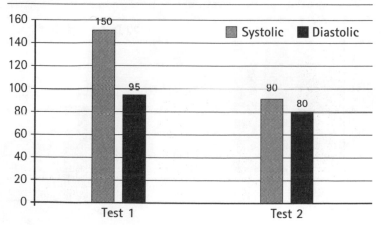

to lower her blood pressure. She follows the 7×6 Heart Plan to achieve these results.

Carmel loves red wine, perhaps a bit too much. She also uses copious amounts of salt in her cooking. As the graph on page 155 depicts, she certainly achieves her goals. Tests before and after twelve weeks of her new low-fat, low-salt, low-alcohol diet show a marked lowering of her blood pressure. The fact that she has lost 8 kilograms of fat during this time is an added bonus, and significantly helps reduce her blood pressure. If you haven't had your blood pressure measured lately, like Carmel, get it done today! Weigh less and be healthy as well.

As the chart below shows, Peter has had his blood pressure measured. Like most men, Peter is adamant that he is fine and there is no need to fuss. As it turns out Peter's blood pressure is quite high and needs urgent attention. There is another

PETER'S BLOOD PRESSURE

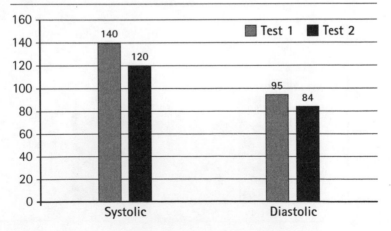

element behind Peter's increased blood pressure. He gets angry and stressed out on numerous occasions. Both anger and stress are risk factors for heart disease and can influence blood pressure. Stress especially can lead to weight gain. Making Peter understand that he could achieve fat loss and lowered blood pressure is quite a task. But he cuts down on beer, fast food, fat and salt and just fourteen weeks later Peter is 10 kilograms lighter and has reduced his blood pressure without medication.

In summary

Some people add only a small amount of exercise into their week, to keep their weight down or to reduce their cholesterol or blood pressure, while others need to do more. If embarking on a program, don't go out and make too many changes too soon. You may put too much pressure on yourself and not adapt to this change. To help you with this, set yourself both short-term and long-term goals.

CHAPTER 7

EATING OUT: TAKING CONTROL

Key messages for this chapter

YOU WILL DISCOVER:

- food eaten at restaurants contains large amounts of fat
- which restaurant and takeaway meals are reasonably low in fat
- how long it takes you to walk off certain foods
- how to keep fat intake to less than 41 grams and 60 grams for men and women respectively

Your secret weapon

The purpose of this chapter is to have a closer look at the foods we eat when we dine out. In putting this information together, I was stunned at the immense fat content of some foods. As a mad football supporter, I used to eat a meat pie or three at a game, as many guys do. As the chart on page 170 shows, each meat pie contains 23 grams of fat. No wonder I used to put on weight; three pies equal 69 grams of fat! This would mean that after every football game I would need to walk for nearly 200 minutes, and cover about 17 kilometres, just to burn off the pies.

We do eat out or purchase takeaway foods a lot more than we did thirty years ago. In Australia we follow trends in both the United States and the United Kingdom, where people are eating more food away from home. For many people, eating at a restaurant means getting their money's worth. This translates into rolling out the door, in other words eating until we're bursting at the seams. When people recommend that we can eat moderate amounts of fat it almost gives us the notion that we can eat what we want. It is in eating out that most of the damage to our fat reserves is done. We justify this by saying, 'But you've got to enjoy life'. For those who love eating out, have a look at the fat content: Italian carbonara, 43 grams; Chinese roast duck in spicy sauce, 60 grams; Thai Panang beef, 47.5 grams; Indian butter chicken, 36 grams; and 100 grams of Mexican corn chips, 34 grams.

When we eat out it is very difficult to discern which foods we should stay away from or eat in smaller amounts for various reasons. For example, your doctor may have told you to cut down on saturated fat, or salt if you have high blood pressure or elevated cholesterol. You may also want to eat 'less fat' when you dine out and explore which foods are reasonably healthy, or the best of the bad so to speak. Dining out without any idea about what is hidden in your meal can be very dangerous. As you will see, some of the foods you love to eat are quite frightening as they are full of fat.

To further coax you into making the right meal decisions when you go out, I have provided an excerpt from the Bilsborough Fat Cost Chart, which shows you the energy cost of each food. How far would you need to walk and for how long after each of these dishes? This is quite staggering but essential for you to understand. I am not criticising these cuisines, but rather trying to find the best dishes that will do as little damage as possible to your health.

Note on servings

All figures listed in the following tables relate to average serving sizes, roughly 200 grams, unless otherwise marked.

Greek restaurants

Greek cuisine is flavoursome and exciting. The meat, primarily lamb, is very tasty and lean. Smaller portions of other dishes are advisable as the fat content can really add up. Beware the dips that always greet you when you arrive at a Greek restaurant. Although very tasty, they are full cream and can really crank up your fat bank.

FOOD	FAT (grams)	WOMEN		MEN	
		WALKING TIME (minutes)	WALKING DISTANCE (kilometres)	WALKING TIME (minutes)	WALKING DISTANCE (kilometres)
taramosalata	19	70	7.3	58	5.4
tzatziki dip (½ cup)	14	59	6.2	48	4.4
olives, black (10)	5	30	3.2	25	2.3
fetta cheese (30 g)	7	36	3.8	30	2.7
calamari fried (5 rings)	17	65	7.2	52	4.8
spanakopita, 1 triangle (cheese & spinach filo pie)	22	81	8.6	64	5.9
moussaka	14	59	6.2	48	4.4
stifado (lamb, potato and onion casserole)	14	59	6.2	48	4.4
souvlaki (2 skewers)	12	50	5.2	41	3.8
galactoburek (custard-filled pastry)	16	62	6.4	50	4.6
kataifi (shredded pastry soaked in honey with nuts)	12	50	5.2	41	3.8

Italian restaurants

The beautiful thing about eating Italian food in Italy is that you get to eat the way the Italians do. They have several small meals, so you never eat a huge bowl of pasta at once. Follow this style of eating in Italian restaurants here, and stay away from the potently rich cream-based foods.

FOOD	FAT (grams)	WOMEN		MEN	
		WALKING TIME (minutes)	WALKING DISTANCE (kilometres)	WALKING TIME (minutes)	WALKING DISTANCE (kilometres)
antipasto	11	48	5	38	3.7
¼ pizza supreme	16	62	6.4	50	4.6
alfredo (small)	24	86	8.9	70	6.2
pasta carbonara	17	69	7.1	55	5
fettuccine marinara	9	41	4.3	34	3.2
pasta pesto	15	59	6.2	48	4.4
spaghetti bolognaise	8	40	4.2	33	3
cannelloni	17	69	7.1	55	5
lasagna	24	86	8.9	70	6.2
gnocchi	10	45	4.7	36	3.5
ravioli	10	45	4.7	36	3.5
chicken cacciatore	15	59	6.2	48	4.4
saltimbocca	28	96	10	80	8.2
veal marsala	21	78	8	62	5.6
osso bucco	19	70	7.3	58	5.4
gelato (4 scoops)	0	0	0	0	0
siena cake	10	45	4.7	36	3.5

Chinese restaurants

The key in Chinese restaurants is to share dishes around the table. Duck is definitely off the menu as it contains too much fat. Pork in plum sauce is a little bit of a concern, so go easy. More rice, preferably steamed with some sweet and sour pork, vegetable stir-fry or beef in black bean sauce, looks like the best option. Saving yourself for a huge feed on a Saturday night at your local Chinese restaurant could be very damaging to your fat intake, especially if you're a duck lover.

FOOD	FAT (grams)	WOMEN		MEN	
		WALKING TIME (minutes)	WALKING DISTANCE (kilometres)	WALKING TIME (minutes)	WALKING DISTANCE (kilometres)
fried noodles (1 cup)	12	50	5.2	41	3.8
fried rice (1 cup)	14	59	6.2	48	4.4
steamed rice (1 cup)	0.3	0	0	0	0
medium spring rolls (3)	17	69	7.1	55	5
beef in black bean sauce	14	59	6.2	48	4.4
beef satay	25.6	88	9.1	72	6.1
beef teriyaki	22	81	8.6	64	5.9
chicken and almonds	19	70	7.3	58	5.4
chicken chow mein	22	81	8.6	64	5.9
crispy chicken	27	95	9.9	75	7.1
lemon chicken	22	81	8.6	64	5.9

continued

FOOD	FAT (grams)	WOMEN		MEN	
		WALKING TIME (minutes)	WALKING DISTANCE (kilometres)	WALKING TIME (minutes)	WALKING DISTANCE (kilometres)
Peking duck	65	292	31.2	234	23
pork in plum sauce	35	162	16.6	130	12.6
sweet & sour pork	18	70	7.3	58	5.4
prawn omelette (½)	32	144	15	115	11.2
prawns in satay sauce	22	81	8.6	64	5.9
satay prawns	17	69	7.1	55	5
vegetable stir-fry	11.5	48	5	38	3.7

Thai restaurants

The mee grob is the loser in the fat grams per serving with a massive 51 grams, and second prize goes to the pad thai with 45.2 grams. Stay away from any dishes with coconut milk or cream – they are particularly bad for cholesterol levels.

FOOD	FAT (grams)	WOMEN		MEN	
		WALKING TIME (minutes)	WALKING DISTANCE (kilometres)	WALKING TIME (minutes)	WALKING DISTANCE (kilometres)
spring roll (150 g)	24	86	8.9	70	6.2
beef panang	47	213	22.3	171	16.6
beef satay with peanut sauce	28	96	10	80	7.2

continued

FOOD	FAT (grams)	WOMEN		MEN	
		WALKING TIME (minutes)	WALKING DISTANCE (kilometres)	WALKING TIME (minutes)	WALKING DISTANCE (kilometres)
thai beef salad	11	48	5	38	3.7
chicken galangal soup with coconut	21	78	8	62	5.6
chicken salad	10	45	4.7	36	3.5
chicken with basil	42	190	19.8	152	14.7
stir-fry ginger chicken	37	167	17.4	133	13
green chicken curry	37	167	17.4	133	13
mee grob	51	229	23.9	184	17.8
pad thai (400 g)	45	202	21.1	162	15.8
spicy fish cakes (150 g)	10	45	4.7	36	3.5
spicy prawn soup (300 g)	3.3	24	2.8	20	1.8
stir-fry prawns with garlic and pepper	24	86	8.9	70	6.2

Indian restaurants

In an Indian restaurant the tandoori chicken is a winner, especially if you ask the chef not to put oil on it before it goes into the tandoor oven. Add a few breads, which always taste good, some lentils, red kidney beans and a potato and pea curry for those needing to consume more legumes, and you almost have a perfect meal. The fat content can be kept down below 30 grams for this meal. The poppadams can be quite fattening, especially if you eat them by the truckload, but tandoori lamb has the most fat with 38.2 grams for a single serve.

FOOD	FAT (grams)	WOMEN		MEN	
		WALKING TIME (minutes)	WALKING DISTANCE (kilometres)	WALKING TIME (minutes)	WALKING DISTANCE (kilometres)
poppadams (2 small)	6	33	3.5	27	2.5
samosas (3)	18	69	7.1	55	5
cucumber raita (20 g)	0.4	0	0	0	0
dhal lentils	8	40	4.2	33	3
kashmiri rice with almonds (100 g)	8	40	4.2	33	3
beef vindaloo	17	69	7.1	55	5
butter chicken	36	162	16.9	129	12.6
chicken tikka	18	69	7.1	55	5
tandoori chicken	14	59	6.2	48	4.4
tandoori lamb chops	38	125	13.3	105	9.5
lamb biryani	28	96	10	80	7.2
lamb korma	19	70	7.3	58	5.4
naan bread (1)	8	40	4.2	33	3
pakora fritters (4)	19	70	7.3	58	5.4
paratha	9	41	4.3	34	3.2
potato pea curry	12	50	5.2	41	3.8
rice, steamed (100 g)	0.2	0	0	0	0
roti (1)	5	30	3.2	25	2.3
spinach curry	33	149	15.5	119	12.6

Vietnamese restaurants

Rice paper rolls packed with vermicelli and lettuce are a refreshing dish, especially with the sharp taste of Vietnamese mint flowing through them. Keep it simple, order steamed rice, stay away from heaps of coconut cream dishes and share your dishes. Another tip is not to have the sauce if you can see there's lots of oil floating on the surface of the dish.

FOOD	FAT (grams)	WOMEN		MEN	
		WALKING TIME (minutes)	WALKING DISTANCE (kilometres)	WALKING TIME (minutes)	WALKING DISTANCE (kilometres)
spring rolls (2 small)	7.6	36	3.8	30	2.7
rice paper rolls	3.3	24	2.8	20	1.8
fish balls (5)	0.5	0	0	0	0
pork balls on skewer	14.2	59	6.2	48	4.4
hot sour soup	8.3	40	4.2	33	3
chicken vermicelli soup	1	18	1.7	15	1.4
rice noodles, steamed	0.7	0	0	0	0
chicken & vegetable curry	18	69	7.1	55	5
ginger chicken stir-fry	18	69	7.1	55	5
pork with lemon grass	17	69	7.1	55	5
beef curry	18	70	7.3	58	5.4
seafood combination	11.4	48	5	38	3.7
prawn and mint salad	7.2	36	3.8	30	2.7
prawns and vegetable stir-fry	14	59	6.2	48	4.4

Lebanese restaurants

The kebabs are very good value, as the fat has a chance to fall off the meat as it is heated. Dishes that contain only plant food are very popular with vegetarians, and for those who are looking for ideas for legumes, there are plenty here. Dishes such as tabbouli and falafel are also good.

FOOD	FAT (grams)	WOMEN		MEN	
		WALKING TIME (minutes)	WALKING DISTANCE (kilometres)	WALKING TIME (minutes)	WALKING DISTANCE (kilometres)
baba ghannosh (½ cup)	24.1	86	8.9	70	6.2
baklava	20.6	75	7.7	60	5.4
hummus (½ cup)	12.1	50	5.2	41	3.8
vine leaves, rice filling (2)	4.6	27	3	23	2.1
lebanese bread	2.5	24	2.8	20	1.8
falafel (1 patty)	7.4	36	3.8	30	2.7
kafta (2)	10.8	48	5	38	3.7
kebbi (1 patty)	10.6	45	4.7	36	3.5
lamb kebab (1 skewer)	7	36	3.8	30	2.7
spinach pie (1 serve)	19.6	70	7.3	58	5.4
tabbouli (½ cup)	12.7	50	5.2	41	3.8

Fast foods

FOOD	FAT (grams)	WOMEN		MEN	
		WALKING TIME (minutes)	WALKING DISTANCE (kilometres)	WALKING TIME (minutes)	WALKING DISTANCE (kilometres)
meat pie	23	83	8.9	66	5.8
Big Mac	24	86	8.9	70	6.2
Cheese Burger	13	52	5.5	44	4.1
Quarter Pounder with Cheese	26	90	9.3	74	6.5
Whopper	39	130	13.6	110	9.9
Bacon Double Cheese Burger	39	130	13.6	110	9.9
Bacon and Egg McMuffin	19	70	7.3	58	5.4
McDonald's Big Breakfast	31	105	11.5	85	7.5
Zinger Burger	17	65	7.2	52	4.8
Chicken Fillet Burger	22	75	8.6	60	5.9
Chocolate Sundae	9	41	4.3	34	3.2
Caramel Sundae	8	40	4.2	33	3
Thick Shake, large	13	52	5.5	44	4.1
Lean Cuisine beef goulash	10	45	4.7	36	3.5
Lean Cuisine chicken carbonara	11	48	5	38	3.7
Lean Cuisine satay lamb	12	50	5.2	41	3.8
Lean Cuisine Thai chicken curry	12	50	5.2	41	3.8
Maggi 2 minute noodles (1 packet)	16	62	6.4	50	4.6

Staple foods

We have seen the vast amounts of fat contained in foods eaten away from home. It follows that the more foods we eat away from home, the more fat we consume. However, other foods we eat often also have a large amount of fat in them. This is why I have provided you with a list of the most commonly eaten foods and their associated energy costs. A common thread of all foods that are high in fat is that they are very low in fibre. You can almost guarantee that the higher the fat content, the lower the fibre content. Use the following tables as a reference for when you're preparing food at home. You'll soon be able to work out which foods you can eat freely, even if you're not following the eating plans, and which you should eat only as an occasional indulgence.

FOOD	FAT (grams)	WOMEN		MEN	
		WALKING TIME (minutes)	WALKING DISTANCE (kilometres)	WALKING TIME (minutes)	WALKING DISTANCE (kilometres)
▶ DAIRY					
butter (1 tablespoon)	15	59	6.2	48	4.4
margarine (1 tablespoon)	15	59	6.2	48	4.4
full-cream milk (1 glass)	10	45	4.7	36	3.5
low-fat milk (1 glass)	0	0	0	0	0
soy-milk (1 glass)	9	41	4.3	34	3.2
plain yoghurt (1 small tub)	8	40	4.2	33	3
cheddar cheese (1 cube)	5	30	3.2	25	2.3
scrambled eggs	15	59	6.2	48	4.4

continued

FOOD	FAT (grams)	WOMEN		MEN	
		WALKING TIME (minutes)	WALKING DISTANCE (kilometres)	WALKING TIME (minutes)	WALKING DISTANCE (kilometres)
▶ GRAINS & CEREALS					
white bread (1 slice)	1	18	1.7	15	1.4
brown bread (1 slice)	1	18	1.7	15	1.4
multi-grain bread (1 slice)	1	18	1.7	15	1.4
pasta (100 g)	1	18	1.7	15	1.4
rice (100 g)	0	0	0	0	0
muffin	11	48	5	38	3.7
muesli bar (full-fat)	4	27	3	23	2.1
croissant	15	59	6.2	48	4.4
▶ MEAT & FISH					
2 lamb chops, grilled, fat on	30	103	10.9	83	7.5
2 lamb chops, grilled, fat trimmed	11	48	5	38	3.7
1 small beef steak, grilled, fat on	26	90	9.4	74	6.5
beef, fat on (¾ cup, diced)	19	70	7.3	58	5.4
beef, fat trimmed (¾ cup, diced)	12	50	5.2	41	3.8
2 sausages, grilled	23	83	8.9	66	5.8
veal schnitzel, fried	39	130	13.6	110	9.9
½ chicken breast, skin on, baked	12	50	5.2	41	3.8
2 bacon rashers, grilled, fat on	13	52	5.5	44	4.1
fish, crumbed and fried	10	45	4.7	36	3.5

continued

FOOD	FAT (grams)	WOMEN		MEN	
		WALKING TIME (minutes)	WALKING DISTANCE (kilometres)	WALKING TIME (minutes)	WALKING DISTANCE (kilometres)
▶ MEAT & FISH – *cont*					
tuna, canned in oil (1 cup)	28	96	10	80	7.2
tuna, canned in brine (1 cup)	5	30	3.2	25	2.3
▶ SNACK FOODS & CONDIMENTS					
peanuts, salted (¼ cup)	21	78	8	62	5.6
potato crisps, (1 packet)	16	62	6.4	50	4.6
peanut butter (1 tablespoon)	13	52	5.5	44	4.1
mayonnaise (1 tablespoon)	7	36	3.8	30	2.7
doughnut, iced	19	70	7.3	58	5.4
rich cream sponge (1 slice)	15	59	6.2	48	4.4
chocolate biscuit	5	30	3.2	25	2.3
Wagon Wheel	8	40	4.2	33	3
chocolate block (6 squares)	8	40	4.2	33	3
jelly babies	0	0	0	0	0
▶ FRUIT & VEG.					
avocado (¼)	14	55	5.9	46	4.2
apple	0	0	0	0	0

continued

FOOD	FAT (grams)	WOMEN		MEN	
		WALKING TIME (minutes)	WALKING DISTANCE (kilometres)	WALKING TIME (minutes)	WALKING DISTANCE (kilometres)
▶ FRUIT & VEG. – *cont*					
banana	0	0	0	0	0
carrot	0	0	0	0	0
potato	0	0	0	0	0
▶ DRINKS					
fruit juice	0	0	0	0	0
lemonade	0	0	0	0	0
red wine	0	0	0	0	0

The fat-cost chart

The Bilsborough Fat Cost Chart really made a huge impact, when it was published in *The Fat-Stripping Diet*, with its ability to analyse excess fat storage. Many people still tell me that when they first started using the chart, they finally felt a sense of reality about what they were doing and eating.

By using the Fat Cost Chart, you can see that the extra fat that the average male and female store needs 100 minutes and 130 minutes of walking time respectively to burn off. In this time 9.5 kilometres and 14 kilometres need to be covered respectively. This is the energy cost of food and it is, as you can see, huge!

The important fact to keep in mind here is that the male body uses about 60 grams of fat every day, while the female body uses around 41 grams. If, for example, Lisa eats 20 grams of fat for a day, then her body needs another 21 grams for energy (41 – 20). This 21 grams comes from her fat stores. If she exercises as well as eating sensibly she will use even more fat from her fat stores.

To remove fat through exercise, as the Bilsborough Fat Cost Chart shows you (see pages 176–177), is very time-consuming. The classic cheese platter can take a few hours to burn up, depending on your idea of moderation. The practical aspect of this chart is not to suggest that you should walk for these times or distances but rather understand that fat takes a very insignificant time to eat but a horrendously long time to remove.

Using the Fat Cost Chart

Using the Bilsborough Fat Cost Chart on pages 176–177 is quite simple. Most of us read the nutritional labels on food packaging to check the amount of fat in each product before we purchase it. Knowing that each gram of fat will correspond to a walking distance and time, you can use the graph to determine roughly how far and for how long you need to walk, given any amount of fat. You can also use this chart to note how much exercise you don't have to do!

When using the chart you will need to add up the total fat grams, the total times and distances for each individual food. Each food has a walking time and distance calculated for it, and each calculation takes into account a 15–20-minute time factor (the time it takes for the body to start using significant amounts of fat). This is the correct way to total up the energy cost of food. Obviously, you don't need to walk for the entire amount of time specified or cover the calculated distance; these graphs simply help you to understand just how much work you need to do to work off your fat intake. It is recommended that you reduce your fat intake in the first instance and then you won't store it.

Reading off how long and how far it takes to burn off individual foods can give you a rough idea of the cost of the food. To find out how much exercise you should do to avoid storing fat, add up your total fat intake for the day, subtract 41 or 60 grams from the total, then calculate your walking distance and time using the chart. This chart can also be used in reverse. For example, if you go for a fast walk for 50 minutes and want to know roughly how much fat you burnt, you simply go to the time axis and read off the corresponding amount of fat. Remember, these values may differ for each individual and they provide a rough guide rather than an exact figure.

How to read the Fat Cost Chart:
1. Go to the amount of fat in a food, for example 15 grams.
2. From this value move up in a straight line until you touch the diagonal.
3. Draw a line across to read the values on the two vertical axes.
4. If the fat consumed is 15 grams, then a man needs to walk for 52 minutes or cover 5 kilometres. For the same amount of fat, a woman needs to walk for 60 minutes or cover 6.8 kilometres.

With this simple method, you can also work out how much fat you will lose if you walk for 45 minutes, for example, or cover 4 kilometres.

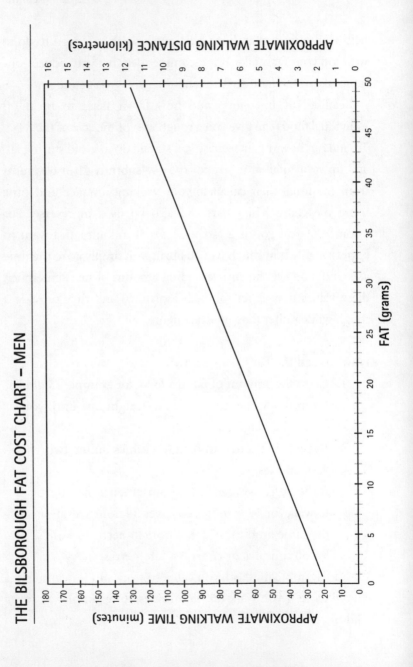

THE BILSBOROUGH FAT COST CHART – MEN

THE BILSBOROUGH FAT COST CHART – WOMEN

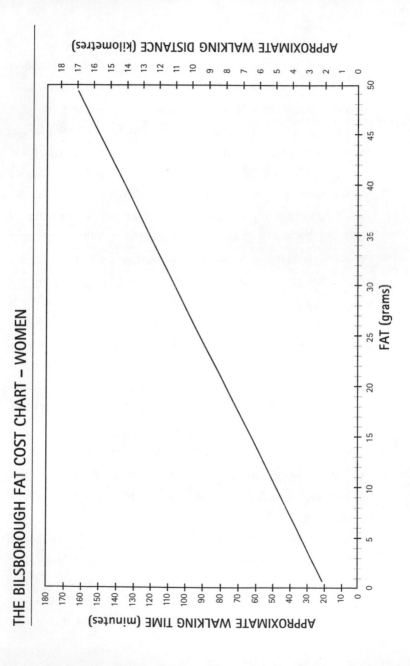

Acknowledgements

Thank you to the following people for their support: fitness trainers Darren Hancock and Mark Wilms from B Personal; Chris Grant, Jason Dowling, Matt McDonald and Ian Martin from Vicfit; Dr Delts – Ian Web; fitness advisor at the South Melbourne Soccer Club Michael Pitchner; Fereti Vasa, the most sought-after personal trainer in Australia; James Podsiadly, the Collingwood gun-rookie; Glen Risley of Spring Foods in South Melbourne; Jeff Olver and Terrence Langendoen.

To Felicity Minchin, the dynamic and inspirational occupational health and fitness guru from BP; the founder of the Fernwood Female Fitness Centres, the wonderful Di Williams; and to the Slimplicity manager Margaret Martin, it has been a privilege to be able to work with people with the same vision. Thank you. Business analysts Freda Miriklis and Andrew Christie; the bubbly Cherie Miriklis of Flowers Vasette; and Patricia Johnson – thank you for all your advice and kind thoughts. And to Paul and Chrissie Velessaris; Josh McKinnon, an amazing guy and good friend; Dr Paul Bergamo; director of the award-winning radio program, 'The Four Diegos Soccer Show', Ralph Barba; RRR's 'Run Like You Stole Something' host and Australian Catholic University senior lecturer in exercise physiology, Justin Kemp.

Thank you to Australia's favourite lady Lillian Frank; Catherine McGill; Karen and Vivien Smith from Vivien's Model Management in Sydney; Danae; Kate Russell; Kate Norton; and Marnie Kayman. A big thank you to Maggie de Chalain from Vivien's Model Management in Melbourne; Mick Case; Glen Moriarty; Dan Thomas; Doug and Maxine Penty; Pauline and Leslie Carrol; Carol; the inspiring Jo Fox; Nick Russian and Cassey Lane; David Medwin;

Tony Di Dio; graphic design whiz Andrew Vargas; Chris Saifert; Lisa Watson; Lisa Mills; and our computer genius Daniel Bilsborough.

To Dr Timothy Crowe from Deakin University, it has been great working with you; and Dr Susan Holt from Sydney University, your work motivates me. My cousin Steve Senn; Mark Barnes; the great philosopher, Graeme Johnson and Stephanie Crouton (the cover girl from *The Fat-Stripping Diet*) from Contemplative Design; Beverley and Berwick Lourensz, who have been wonderful friends for such a long time; Colin Delutis – the great one; Carl and Sandra Clark; Dad and Lin; Mum and Neal.

I must thank three people from Penguin with whom I have worked closely: my publicist Melissa Roos, who has always been so much fun; Kirsten Abbott, my editor, whose understanding, hard work and visionary intuition have had a huge influence on the development of this book; and my publisher Clare Forster – thanks for the belief, support and hard work over the past few years. Thank you all also for helping make *The Fat-Stripping Diet* a number one bestseller.

Thank you to Dr David Cameron Smith from Deakin University for his guidance and help whenever I have needed it. Not only was he a fantastic lecturer and research scientist, but also a good friend and awesome to work with. My brother, Johann, who is the co-director of B Personal, has also been a source of strength and inspiration, and is an exceptional exercise scientist. And finally, thanks to my wife Fiona, who is also my walking and jogging partner, my gym partner, a gourmet chef and the beautiful cover girl of *7 Days to Strip Fat Forever*.

INDEX